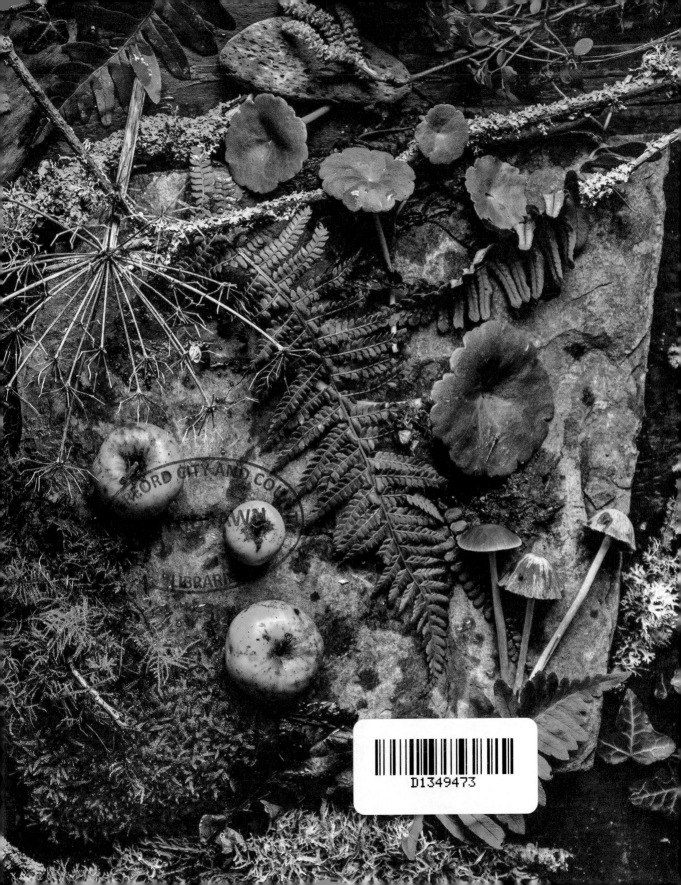

fforest

fforest
Being, doing & making in nature

Sian Tucker

K

An Hachette UK Company
www.hachette.co.uk

First published in Great Britain in 2019
by Kyle Books, an imprint of Kyle Cathie Ltd
Carmelite House,
50 Victoria Embankment,
London, EC4Y 0DZ
www.kylebooks.com

ISBN: 978 0 85783 591 8

Distributed in the US by Hachette Book Group,
1290 Avenue of the Americas, 4th and 5th Floors,
New York, NY 10104

Distributed in Canada by Canadian Manda Group,
664 Annette St., Toronto, Ontario, Canada M6S 2C8

Editorial Director: Judith Hannam
Editorial Assistant: Isabel Gonzalez-Prendergast
Designer: The Department of Small Works
Photographer: Finn Beales
Production: Lisa Pinnell

A Cataloguing in Publication record for this
title is available from the British Library.

Printed and bound in China.

10 9 8 7 6 5 4 3 2 1

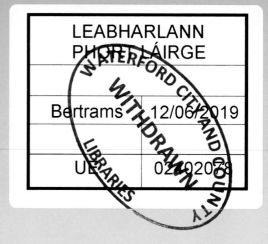
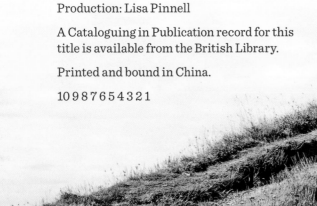

Contents

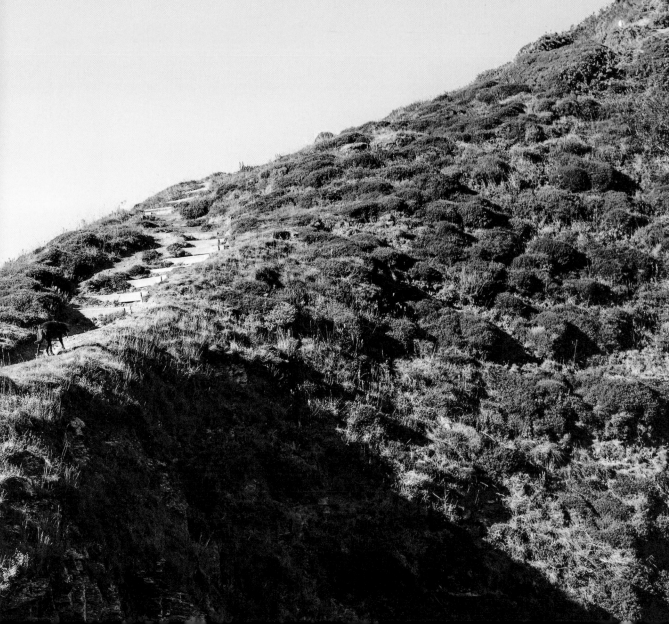

There is another alphabet, whispering
from every leaf, singing from every river,
shimmering from every sky.
Dejan Stojanović

fforest is the name of our 200-acre farm
set on high land surrounded by ancient oak
woods on the edge of the Teifi Gorge.

This farm has been called fforest for centuries, probably since the
fourteenth century. The land lies between two very old castles,
one in the small town of Aberteifi (Cardigan), the other in the
village of Cilgerran. There is evidence of there having been an
Iron Age settlement here too. It is a beautiful part of unspoilt land
on the far west of Wales very close to a stunning coastline of slate
rocks and cliffs with secluded coves and beaches.

James and I moved to fforest from London with our young family
of four boys in the middle of winter 2005. Arriving at the Winter
Solstice seemed like a good idea at the time, as the days would
soon be getting longer, but with sunset at just after four o'clock it
was impossible to be outside after school to play for quite a while.

Every day we notice the light on the trees, through the clouds and
on the sea, and the seasons passing, little by little. These things
feed our souls. Our favourite thing to do is to spend the day with
family and friends. We walk over the cliff tops or pootle by boat
across the sea to a secret beach and then set up a camp, collecting
driftwood, making a fire and diving for spider crabs. We then cook
over the flames and eat. We swim, we paddle and play games till
sunset, then we head for home. This is as good as it gets. Cooking
and eating, laughing and being outside with those you love is
blissful for the body, for the heart and for the mind.

I have known this part of Wales all my life, but moving from central London to settle here full time and start creating fforest was a whole new exciting adventure. Over the years we have slowly been creating a place where living, playing, inspiration, adventure and learning can happen in the beauty of the great outdoors, by sleeping under canvas and listening to nature. We came full of ideas of how to create a feeling of community, although we had very little experience in hospitality. It was in April 2007 that we bravely opened the doors to fforest farm and the journey began to where we are today.

This book is an extension of the life we have created at fforest. It is designed to inspire you to get outdoors, to try new skills, to be comfortable with exploring nature, and to understand a little more of the world that surrounds us and the pleasures and benefits it can give us. It is surprising how much we can gain just by being outside, and how many ways there are to fully embrace the outdoors, from walking in the dark with only the light of the moon and the stars to guide us, to swimming in wild water and lighting a fire.

This is not a survival manual, or maybe it is — for surviving the deficits of modern life by learning to be still, to engage with nature, to do things that would have been second nature to us only a generation or two ago, to rediscover simple pleasures. I hope it inspires you to learn new skills and discover, or rediscover, what it is to be outside.

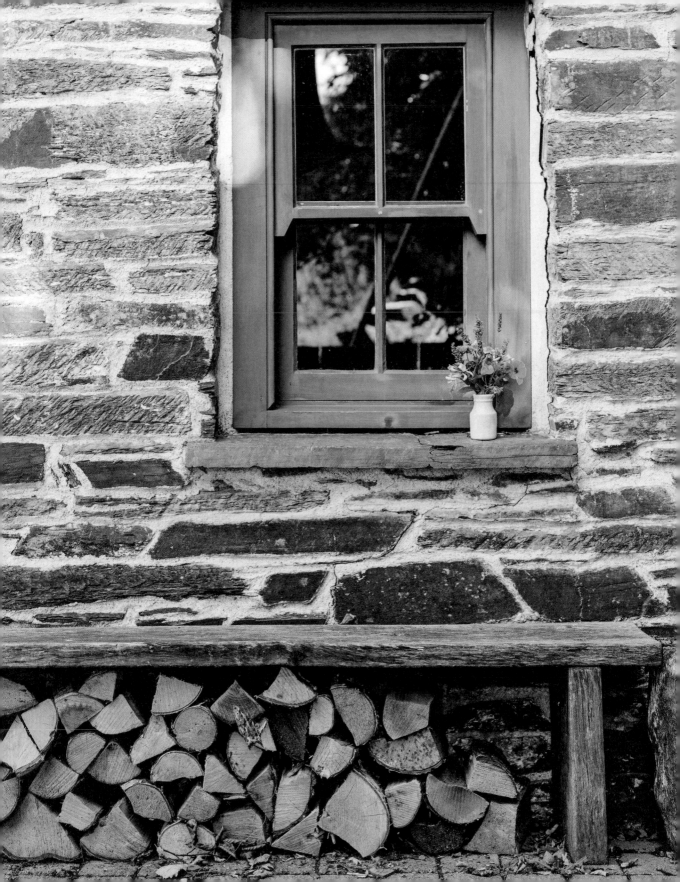

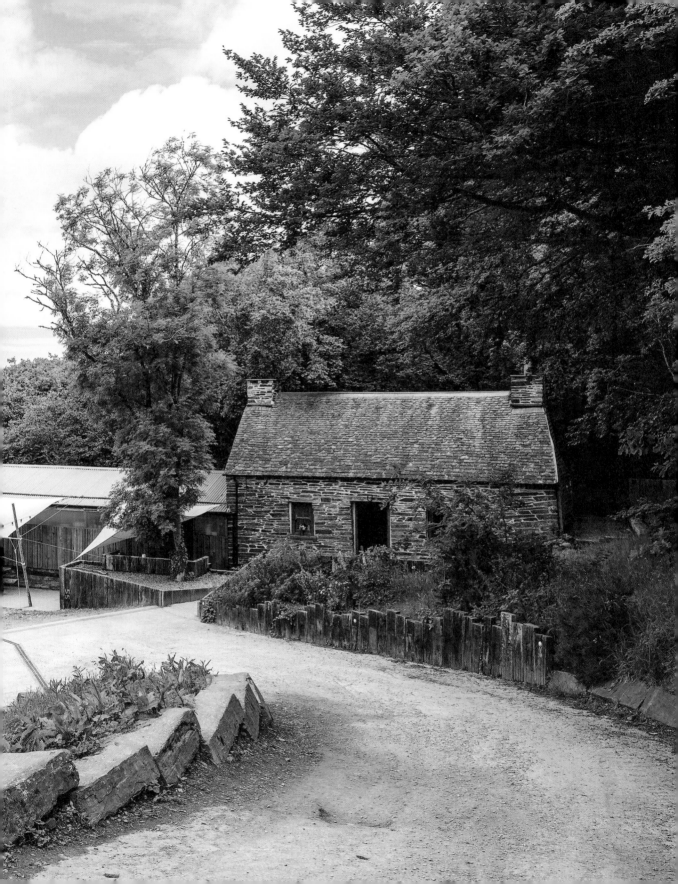

Nature does not hurry,
yet everything is accomplished.
Lao-tzu

fforest is made up of a thousand simple details, lighting fires, flickering candles, picking flowers, eating a simple breakfast together, cooking outside, living, playing and learning in a beautiful, natural environment with minimum consumption and minimum of means.

When guests arrive, we like to give them time to settle after their long journey. We invite them to leave their car in the car park and walk up to the lodge along the tree-lined footpath, through a small coppice wood of willow and hazel, to a welcoming cup of tea with a view over the meadows. We like to encourage them to take some time to sit, decompress and relax, to gain a feeling of comfort in their new surroundings, to begin to feel at home, and to have a happy heart.

fforest is the simplest and purest of things all wrapped up in a magical setting. At fforest 'simple' is both a way and a place. It's where you get to once you pause, wind down, be properly still. Only then can you become immersed in your surroundings, the place we call simple. Only when you stop and listen can you notice the little things and find joy in tiny details — the rustling of leaves in the breeze, the flicker of flames in the fire, tiny wild flowers, birdsong, moonlight.

Working closely with Mother Nature has taught us to respect and understand her ways, rhythms and cycles. By finding time to tune in to the pace of the natural world, grounding ourselves and letting our minds be still, we will learn to appreciate the rich diversity of where we are.

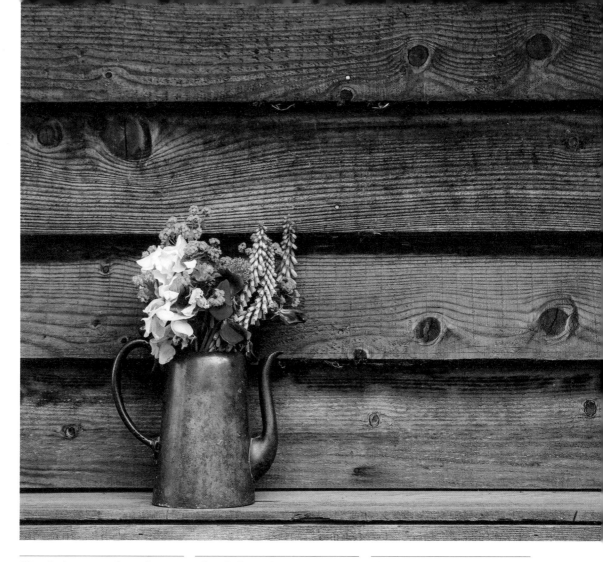

Simple is savouring where you are, indulging your senses and appreciating the seasonal changes. As you walk through ancient woodlands, wild meadows or along coastal footpaths, listen to the wind whispering in the trees, the birds singing and the stream gurgling. Stop and smell the earth, notice the rain-washed leaves, feel the tall grasses as you brush past.

Simple is caring. It's taking care of our environment. It's conservation, recycling, reusing and nurturing nature. It's feeding the birds and attracting the bees. It's eating well, wisely and healthily, shopping locally and growing your own vegetables. Whether it's in polytunnels, as we have at fforest, or in a few pots on a window ledge, they will have a magical taste, the taste of care and nurture.

Simple is daydreaming, mind wanderings and brain drifting. It's a point between being here in the now and in a dream land. It's being quiet, feeling comfortable in silence and with others in silence, of not feeling the need to talk. It's creating a gap to calm our thoughts and empty our minds. Giving yourself just a few moments of silence and a few deep breaths can release tension in the body and mind.

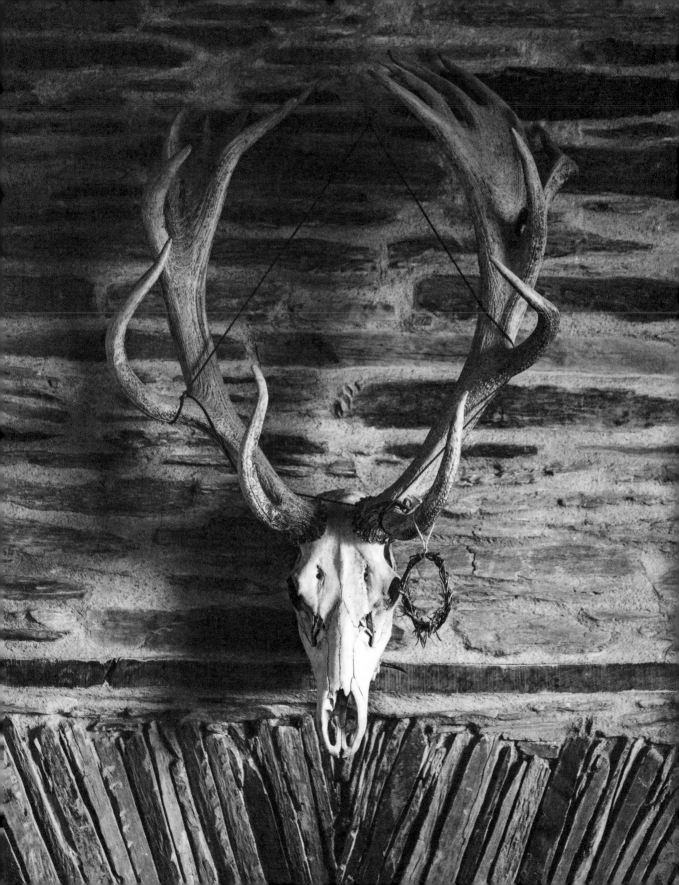

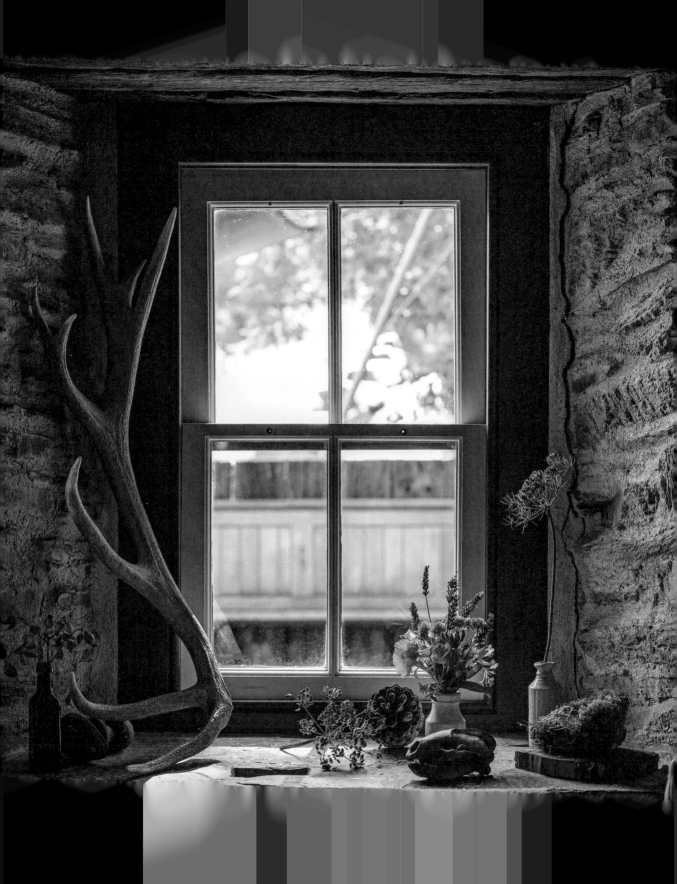

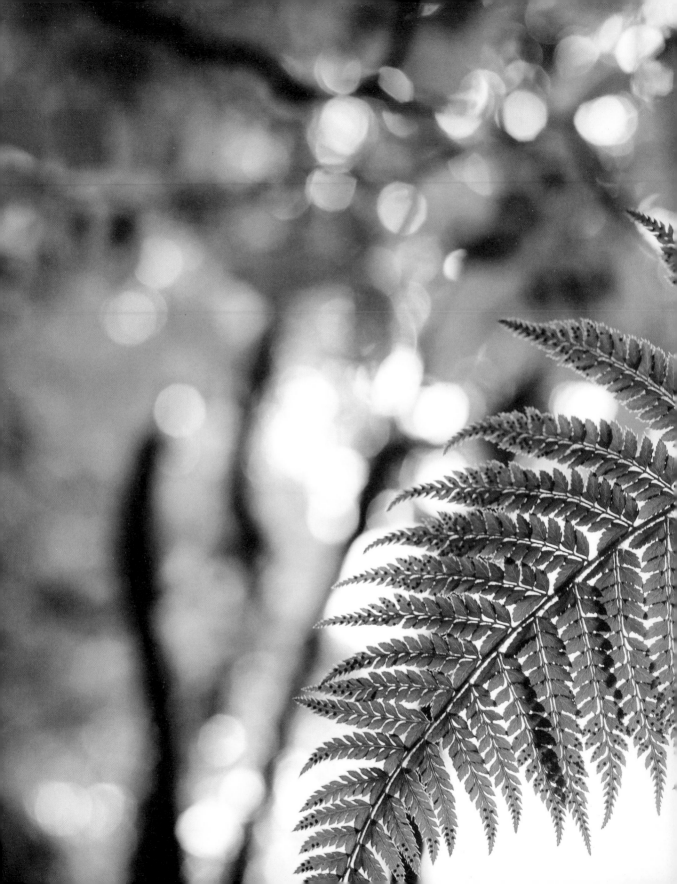

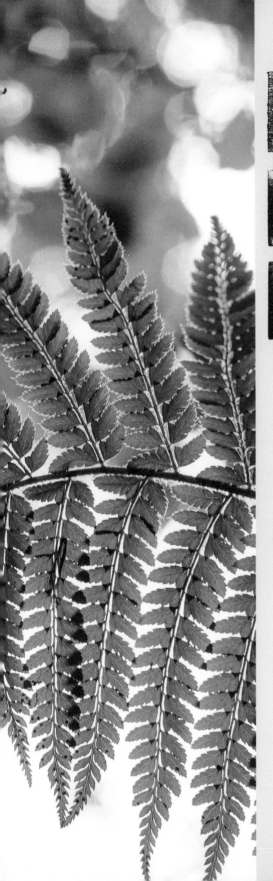

BEING
IN
NATURE

Nature itself is the best physician.
Hippocrates

Not so many years ago most of us lived off
the land, walking everywhere or riding a
horse, spending most of our waking hours
outdoors in close contact with nature and
the changing seasons.

Until recently, children were told to play outside until suppertime,
and as a result had so many positive relationships with nature
and adventures and stories to tell.

Every day, morning and evening, we walk our dogs on the beach.
We are lucky. When I stand there, staring across the horizon into
the far distance, the salty sea wind blowing through my hair,
waves crashing against the rocks, the sea lapping and foaming
onto the sand, I am struck by the immensity of nature and always
feel so much better, happier and clearer headed after drinking in
its sounds and smells.

A growing body of research tells us that being outside is good
for us. The shared experience of being in nature, of working and
playing outside, of sitting in the dark around a fire, of whittling
a stick, is conducive to our sharing thoughts and ideas that we
wouldn't necessarily want to talk about at any other time. Being
in touch with the wild encourages us to connect with each other,
strengthens family bonds and helps create community. Humans
are social animals and we need to interact with each other.

Increasing urbanisation and the rise in popularity of social media has meant that people go outside less and less. It is almost as if they are afraid of nature, fearful of being swallowed up by it, of being alone in it. But when we embrace the mystery and beauty of nature and feel its slow pulse, there tends to be a deep connection, a calmness, a joy, a trust in life, a spiritual wellbeing, even healing. This is something that only you can experience yourself. Only you can take time to discover the power of nature and the awe and wonder of the natural elements.

When we are outside we naturally become more active. This releases the endorphins that make us feel so much better. Exercise taken outside in green spaces has greater health benefits than exercise taken indoors. Nature has an incredible ability to seep inside us, to provide calm, comfort and serenity.

So take a moment to slow down. Sit in a garden. Go for a walk in a park. Listen to the birds. Cycle along a river or go to the sea. Being outside can boost our energy and mood, it can help us unclutter our minds and connect to ourselves, to feel more active and alive. When you sit by a stream, listen to the water gliding over smooth, mossy boulders, breathe in the mild, still air smelling of fresh green and damp earth. When you walk through a sea of swaying meadow grasses, listen to the bees buzzing, watch a buzzard swooping. Seeing the sun rise or set, watching the clouds float by, all these things will lighten your mood and make you feel happier and more connected to the world around you.

Live in the sunshine, swim in the sea,
drink the wild air.
Ralph Waldo Emerson

Scandinavia seems to have many of the answers for a good and happy life. According to UN rankings, Denmark is the happiest country on Earth and Norway is the second most content.

Friluftsliv **is a Norwegian word that translates as 'free air life'.** This concept encapsulates a way of life powered by nature, of being present in the great outdoors, of how by spending time outside we learn of the power of nature and its ability to induce deep and spiritual feelings.

It's an expression of how precious life is and how, in order to relate to the more than human world that we live in, we must remind ourselves that we, too, are connected to the circle of life and belong to nature.

The word *Friluftsliv* first appeared in the work of the Norwegian poet Henrik Ibsen in 1859. It can be used to describe any outside activity, from hiking a mountain, to fishing in the river, lake or sea, foraging and picking berries in the hedgerows, having a picnic with friends or going for a walk or a bike ride. It's about enjoying being in nature whatever the weather, winter or summer, day or night, rain or shine, mud or snow. It's about listening, looking and feeling nature's rhythm, patterns and soul-soothing harmony.

Many factors contribute to building a healthy and happy society, but encouraging awareness and interest in the outdoors is central to the Norwegian way of life.

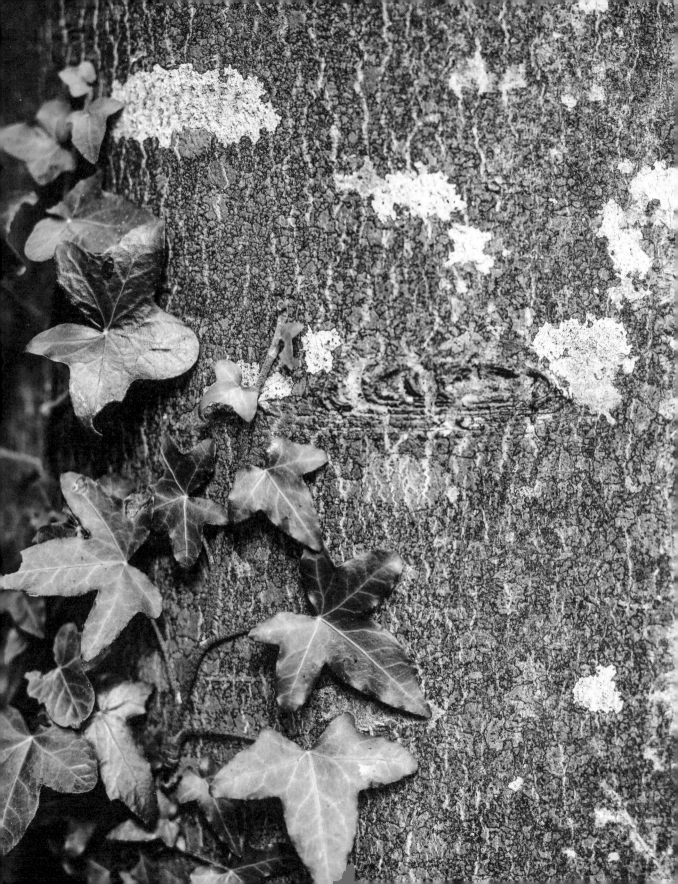

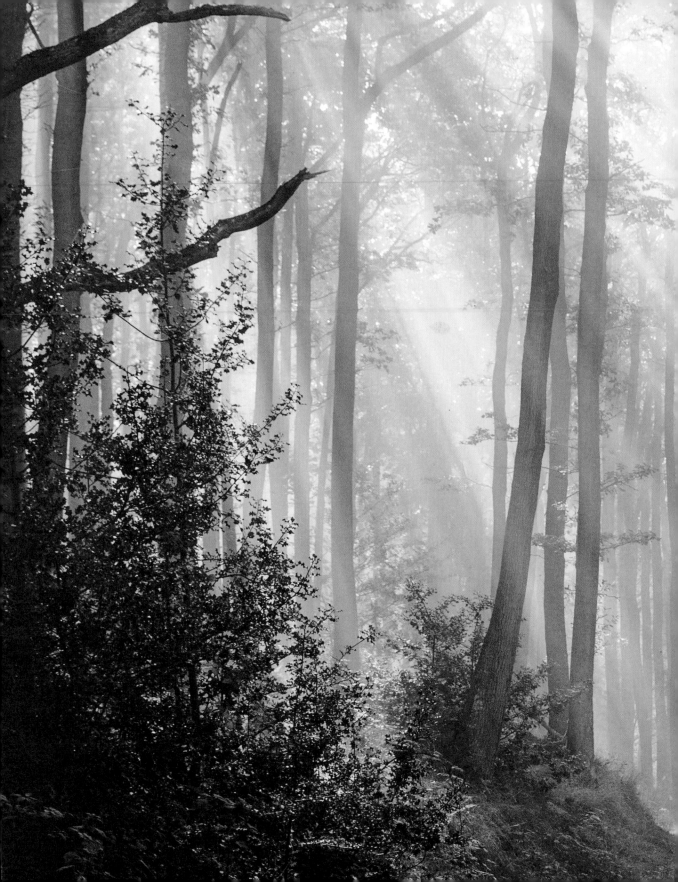

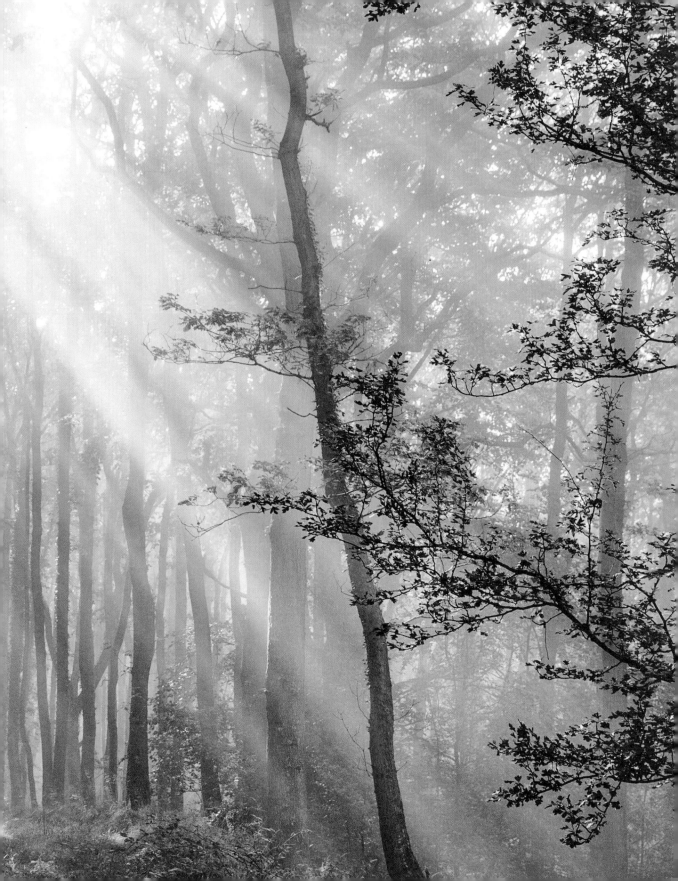

Colour all around us

Mere colour, unspoiled by meaning, and unallied with definite form, can speak to the soul in a thousand different ways.
Oscar Wilde

Colour has an impact on our sense of wellbeing. It can influence our mood, energise or calm us, heal or irritate. It can affect our sleep patterns, digestion and appetite. In nature, colour is all around us, constantly changing with the light and seasons. Each day offers something different. We can look and take delight in how colour plays on flora and fauna, and be inspired by the incredible palette created, a palette that can be vibrant, strong, soft, subtle, warm or cold.

Green is the colour of Mother Nature and of the Earth. It represents balance, harmony, peace, comfort, fertility and growth, and has a calming effect on both our mind and body, easing us from anxiety, depression and nervousness. Just having plants and fresh flowers in the home can have a soothing effect.

Blue is the colour for health and holistic thought, for dreams and daydreams. It refreshes, cools and calms us, offering peace and tranquility; feelings we experience viewing a clear blue sky on a sunny day.

Red is the colour of vitality, courage and self-confidence. A great energiser, it excites us, increasing our heart rate. It's the colour of fire, blood, berries and roses, warming and awakening us physically. Red is also associated with passion, love, sex, heat, power and adventure.

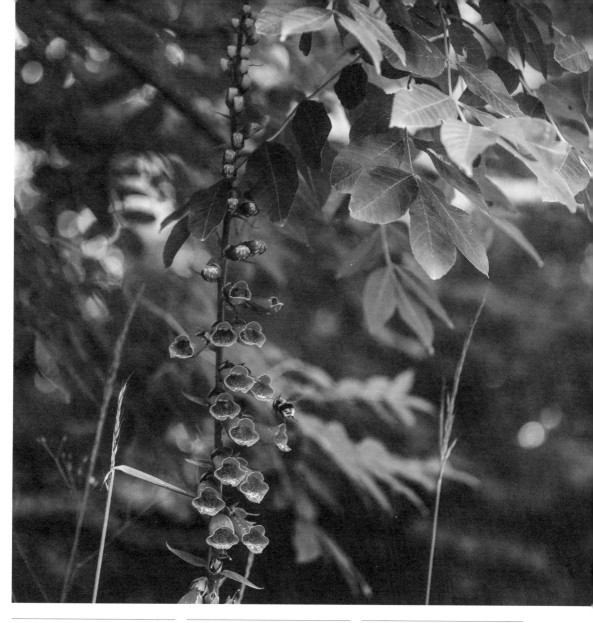

Orange is the colour of happiness, confidence, joy and wisdom; it stimulates mental enlightenment and greater understanding. It also removes inhibitions and strengthens our appetite for life. It's the warm glow of embers, a beautiful sunset, the golden leaves of autumn.

Yellow is the colour of life itself — of the big, bright fiery ball in the sky, of vitality and cheerfulness. Yellow is also the colour of clarity and curiosity. It helps relieve depression and increase self-esteem. It's the colour that awakens and inspires the mind, improves memory, stimulates the nervous system and energises us.

White is all colour in perfect harmony and balance. It's the colour of purity, of calm, cleanliness, hope, simplicity, elegance and innocence. It awakens the spirit. It's the colour of fluffy clouds, of frost and of ice and snow.

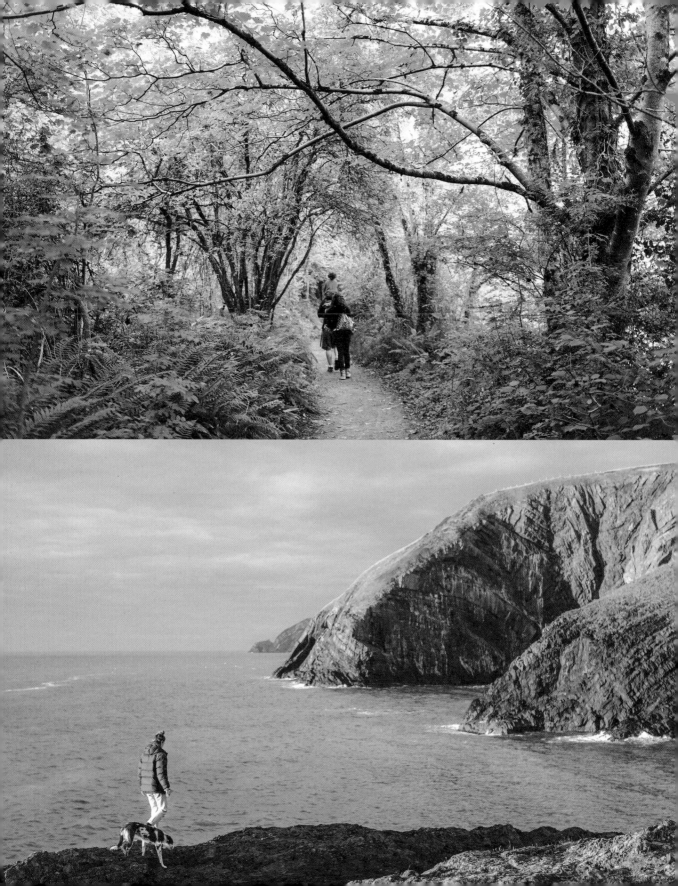

Walking

Nature is painting for us, day after day, pictures of infinite beauty if only we have the eyes to see them.
John Ruskin

Rambling, ambling, hiking, trekking, tramping, trudging, roaming, stomping, sauntering, wandering — there are endless words to describe good old-fashioned walking, but whatever you call it, the benefits are immense. The rhythm of walking echoes our beating heart, the stepping motion re-jigs our brain, it clears our minds and encourages thought. It allows us to feel the flow of our blood, our breath and our step, stimulates a warmth in our heart and gives us a rosy cheek glow.

At fforest, we organise all sorts of activities around and about. But when does normal life become an activity? Is going for a walk normal life or an activity? I don't think it's helpful to 'package' life in this way. Either James or I often take our guests on a walk, part of which goes through the farm, and part through the adjoining nature reserve and along the Teifi Gorge.

We might have 6 people or 20, and ages 3 to 73. At a leisurely pace, the walk takes about 90 minutes, but is tough enough in patches for everyone to know they've had some exercise. It's a beautiful, life-enhancing walk, encompassing the river, landscape, wildlife, history and dragons. What we've learnt from doing it is that people get a lot out of a little. OK, it's a great walk, but the magic is in the learning of little things, the ebb and flow of the conversation, the way the smaller kids don't notice the harder climbs, the way everyone knows everyone else just a little bit better at the end. The sense of a shared small achievement isn't something that happens indoors.

Walking in the dark

It was only once we were living here, in this rural part of West Wales, that we realised that London, like all other big cities, never really gets properly dark. And because you never get to feel the true sense of the darkness of long winter nights in urban areas — where the streets have lights, huge office towers are always lit and the climate is modified by the density of the buildings — our ability to feel the day, night and seasons is fractured.

Most of us are afraid of being out in the dark, of walking in the countryside in the gloom of the dusky shadows and silvery glows, the not quite seeing. A city late at night has its own dangers, but a determined-and-with-purpose speed walk will get you home fast and fine. A walk in the woods, through a field or across a deserted beach on a cloudy night without a moon is DARK. The sort of darkness that has an animal quality, like a living thing. All your other senses — hearing, touch, smell — become heightened and alert, making up for your weakened sight.

People have been walking across these fields at fforest from one place to the other for thousands of years. When darkness closes in at the end of the day, blurring the boundaries of space and distance, smells of dew and damp earth and grasses change, and when walking in the dark sometimes our imagination can get the better of us... inventing, hearing, seeing things.

It best to use your torch sparingly, to let your eyes adjust to the dark and to rely on your ears and nose to help you find your way around. Every time we go out into the dark there is always a nervousness about the unknown and not being able to see properly, like when you go into the deep sea, but as you become accustomed to your surroundings, you can slowly physically connect with the blackness. Once you have done so, you can listen out for snuffles of night animals.

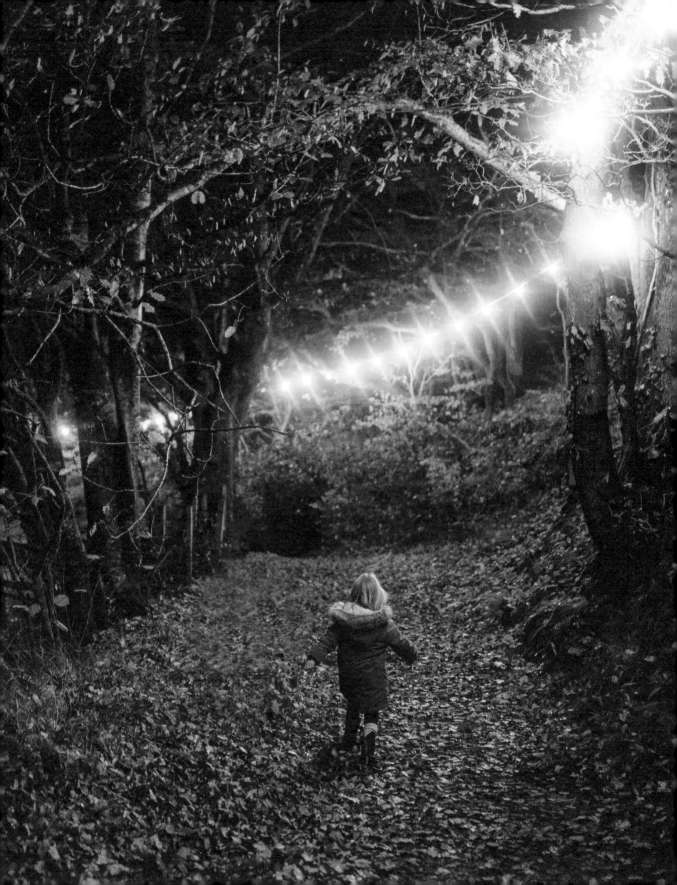

Forest bathing

Walk tall as the trees, live strong as the mountains, be gentle as the spring winds, keep the warmth of the summer sun in your heart and the great spirit will always be with you.
Native American proverb

Forest bathing means to 'bathe' all your senses in the beauty and the nature of the woods. It's not a bath nor a swim, it's not a hike either, but a gentle walk in the woods, slowing right down to tune into all your senses.

Stand and feel the ground beneath you, walk slowly, breathe calmly and deeply, listen to the silence. Take in the smell of the earth, notice the rustle of the leaves in the canopy above, the light glimmering, twinkling, shimmering through the leaves, shadows dancing on the bark of the trees.

Going into the woods to be immersed is not about the physical exercise of getting somewhere as quickly as you can, but more a woodland meditation. In Japan they call this *shinrin-yoku* 'nourished by nature'.

Not so long ago, when we were more connected to nature, we lived by its rhythms and by the natural push and pull of the seasons. Nature was in our blood and we spent much of our time outside working with it.

We walked everywhere and would have noticed even the smallest seasonal changes. We probably pondered and daydreamed too. But now our lives have become so fast paced we rush past without looking. We are here and there, doing loads of stuff and are distracted by technology, travelling in cars, trains and buses, spending more and more time indoors, increasingly disconnected from nature and the outdoors.

Scientific studies in Japan have shown time spent immersed in nature is hugely beneficial, particularly if it is spent surrounded by the gentle beauty of trees, stilling our minds, calming our thoughts and slowing down our breathing. Breathing in the forest air, rich with oxygen and earthy, woody aromas, combined with taking time to contemplate the beauty of nature, results in increased mental wellbeing, reduced stress levels and blood pressure and boosts our immune systems.

The wild is in us, it is in our bones, it is in our blood, it is a part of who we are.

When you are next in a woodland there are things you can do to calm your mind and stimulate your imagination. They are not things you have to do alone, you can go in a small group, but make sure you find space on your own for a while.

The woods will always be your friend, trees are good listeners. If you can't get to a forest, go to a park where there are trees and have some quiet contemplation.

Leave your phone behind, so you can be fully present to absorb and connect to yourself and where you are. Make sure you give plenty of time to open yourself to the ancient woodland whispers.

Walk slowly, breathe deeply, take time to explore your surroundings. Touch, feel and smell the earth. Sit, be aware of your solitude, be truly in what is around you and enjoy the moment.

Absorb everything. Notice the colours and shapes of nature. Hug a tree and feel the slow energy, feel quiet, feel calmed.

Stand still in silence, be calm, there is no rush. Slowly welcome the gifts of the forest. I know it is often hard to be still and you might feel self-conscious, maybe even afraid to stand alone, a small speck amongst the tall trees, a little dot of mankind on this big spinning rock called Earth. But standing beneath a majestic tree, with all its gathered wisdom, something so old, so calming and quietly energising, the home to so many woodland creatures, as well as lichen, fungi and moss, is magical.

Immerse yourself in your senses and notice the tiny details of your surroundings, the gnarly roots growing firm, strong and deep, anchoring into the ground, the tangled vines climbing up smooth and twisted trunks, a forest floor of soft, paper-thin leaves, shafts of light, pine needles, pine cones, a carpet of bluebells, a whiff of wild garlic in the air.

Ask yourself how it makes you feel to be surrounded by nature. Are you comfortable in this space around you, what did you notice? Maybe there are secrets you would like to throw up into the wind to be blown away. Maybe there are promises you wish to keep and take home with you.

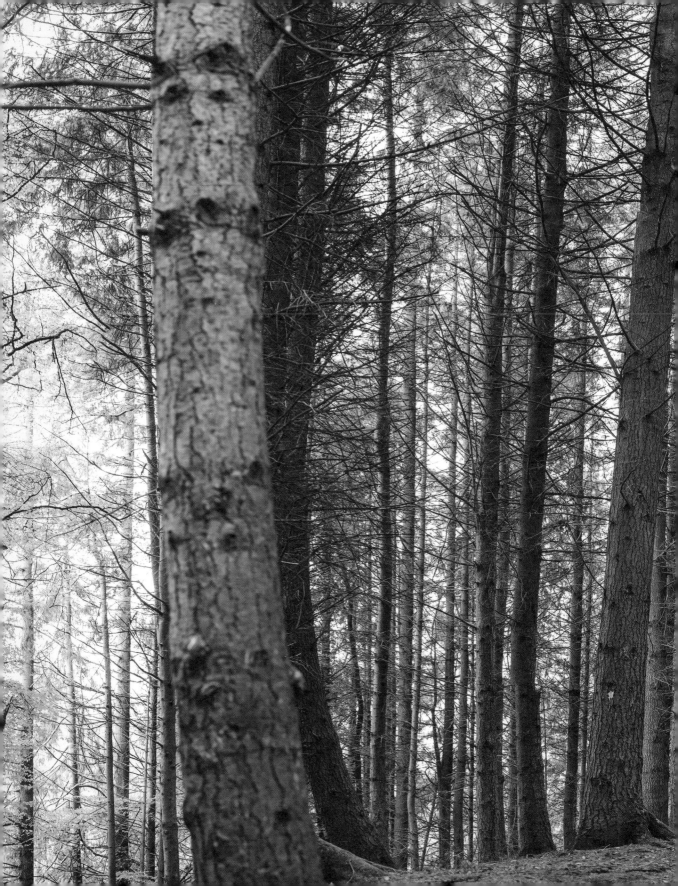

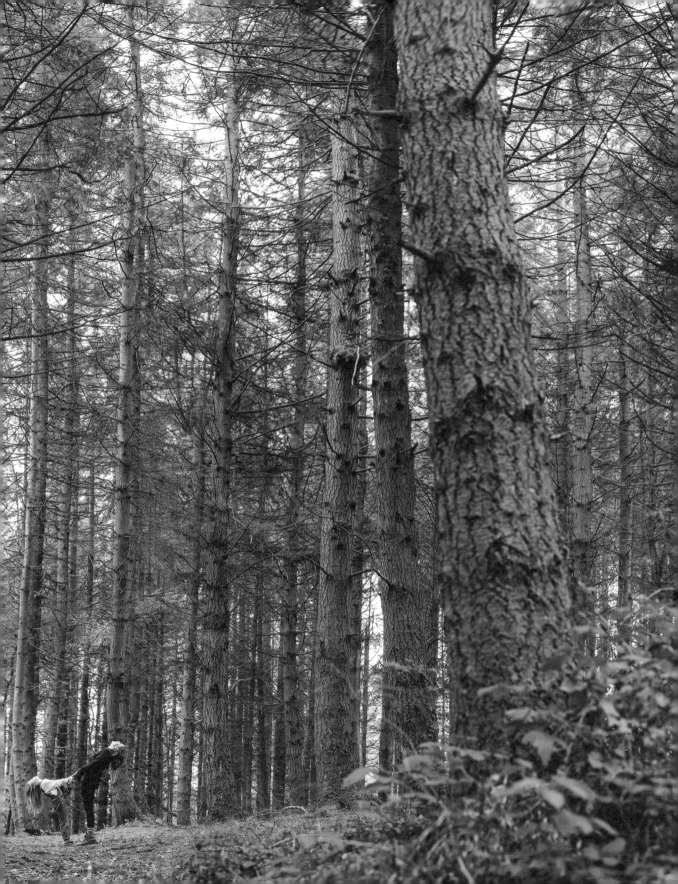

Daydreaming

The quieter you become,
the more you are able to hear.
Rumi

When we find ourselves zoning out, when our minds are wandering and drifting off into space like a fluffy, floaty cloud and we are seemingly not getting anything much done, we have to ask, is daydreaming a waste of time?

James is especially guilty of sitting in his own little world looking like he isn't doing anything much at all. Research has shown that he is not alone and it is common to spend up to half of our waking hours daydreaming. Daydreaming can be useful, however. There are benefits to be had from whiling away the day, including helping to improve memory and attention span. Mind wandering and mind drifting increase creative connections in the brain and can help lower blood pressure, thereby reducing anxiety and relieving stress, helping us to become happier and healthier.

By taking a mini brain break from a task, our unconscious mind is free to become active, to wander into the past or imagine the future, exploring, collecting and reconnecting many bits of gathered information together, forming new thoughts and ideas, new creative solutions, new beginnings. So daydream on, drift away...

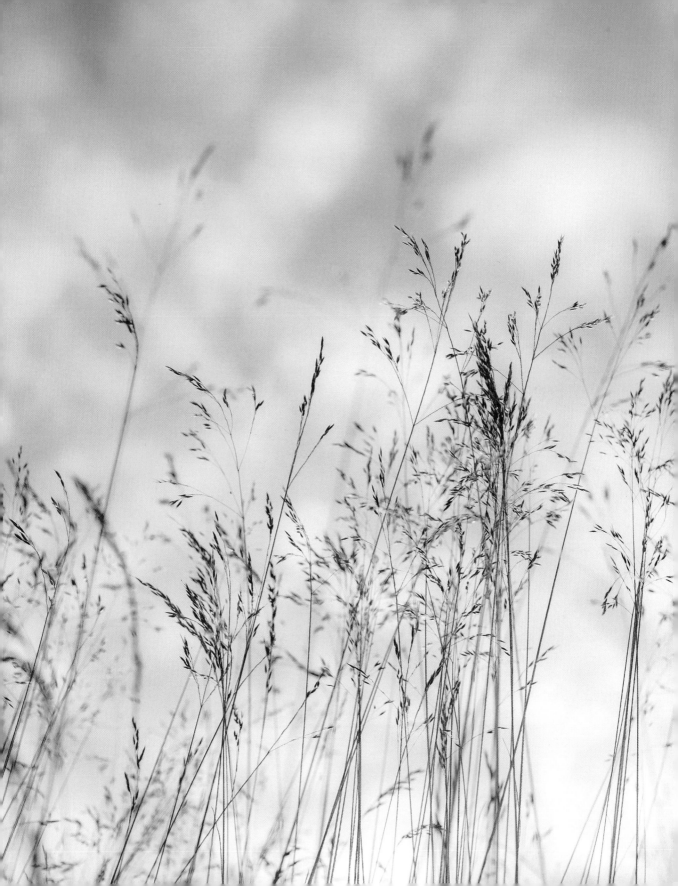

Cloud-gazing

Rest is not idleness, and to lie sometimes on the grass under trees on a summer's day, listening to the murmur of the water, or watching the clouds float across the sky, is by no means a waste of time.
John Lubbock

Life would be so dull if we had only clear blue skies and sunshine every day without a threatening cloud in sight. Earth is a lush, watery, blue-green planet, our life depends on water and we are watery beings. Without water, Earth would be cloudless, there would be no rain, no plants, no sea, no rivers and no life.

Clouds are the magic show of the sky. Continually moving, appearing and disappearing, they can be rolling, fluffy, fleecy, floaty, feathery, blobby, wispy and ethereal, as well as milky, misty, foggy, gloomy, dense, dark, brooding, stormy, threatening and ominous. Contemplating the why, the how, the where do they go is endlessly fascinating. At fforest, living as we do on the edge of the Gulf Stream, where hot air from the south moves up over the sea to the north, continuously bringing endless watery clouds and weather, we spend a lot of time talking and thinking, looking and wondering what the sky is going to give us each day.

Gazing up at the sky will fill you with awe and wonder. You'll be humbled at the sheer beauty of our world, the skies above it and the constantly moving and floating shapes that filter the light and shift the colours.

Here in the UK, where we get alot of rain, clouds can be viewed negatively, 'a cloud on the horizon' means something threatening or bad is going to happen.

Across the world, clouds can induce very different feelings. In Iran, clouds are considered lucky. It is a blessing to say 'your sky is always filled with clouds.' Rain dances were common to many cultures in areas of drought and were done to encourage clouds and rain to water the land for the crops.

Hamlet	Do you see yonder cloud that's almost in shape of a camel?
Polonius	By the mass, and 'tis like a camel, indeed.
Hamlet	Methinks it is like a weasel.
Polonius	It is backed like a weasel.
Hamlet	Or like a whale?
Polonius	Very like a whale.

Hamlet, Act 3, Scene 2
William Shakespeare

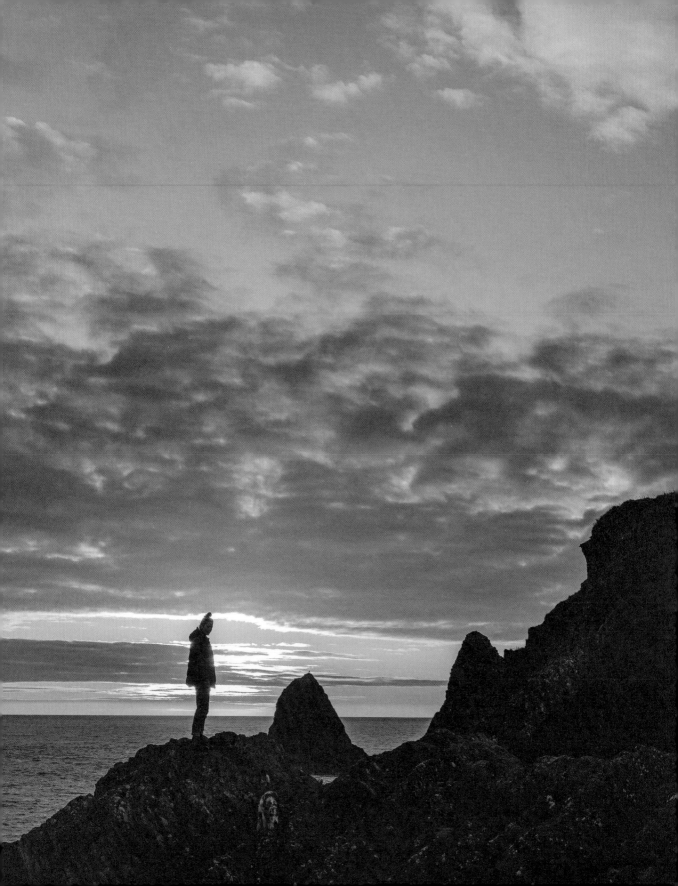

A simple guide to the clouds

There's no such thing as bad weather, only unsuitable clothing. Alfred Wainwright

Cumulus clouds are the fair weather clouds that look just like the ones children draw: rounded, puffy, brilliant blobs of cotton-wool fluff on a sunny day. They tend to have a flattish bottom, appear late morning, billow across the sky during the day, then fade away towards evening.

Stratus clouds are often filled with a light misty drizzle. They hang low in the sky as flat, featureless, dull and dreary uniform layers of greyish cloud that resemble the fog that hugs the horizon.

Cirrus clouds are thin, white, feathery, delicate, wispy strands of cloud made from ice crystals that streak across the sky, swept along by high winds. They form above 6,000 metres (20,000 feet) and typically occur in fair weather. When they gather and clutter it can mean storms are brewing.

Nimbus clouds are the bearers of rain. Large and greyish black in colour, they're drifting and spreading blankets of cloud hanging low across the sky, carrying huge amounts of water that comes down as rain, rain, rain.

Cumulonimbus clouds grow and bulge like cauliflower florets. They tower high into the sky, their bottoms dark, flat and hazy and full of water. They bring the promise of severe weather, hail, thunder rolls, lightning crashes, pouring rain and storms.

Thunder and lightning

Storms are a demonstration of the power of nature, both terrifying and mesmeric. You occasionally hear of someone being struck by lightning, but the incidence of it happening is very rare. Nevertheless, if you are caught outside in a storm keep away from open areas, don't take shelter under a solitary tall tree, avoid water (so don't go swimming) and make sure you are not holding anything metal. All these things act as conductors, making you more likely to get struck. Instead, take refuge in a building or car. Try counting the seconds in between the lightning strikes and thunder claps... one thousand, two thousand... this helps to establish how far away the strikes are. It's roughly a kilometre (3,300 feet) for each second.

Thunderstorms are dramatic events, so it's not surprising that they cause excitement and also fear. Animals and small children are especially fearful of the loud claps and rolling, growling rumbles that echo through the air, sending them to hide for cover.

It is good to know, therefore, that thunderstorms can be beneficial. During a storm the air is purified and negative ions are created in abundance. These are anything but negative when it comes to our health. Studies show that breathing in air that is rich in negative ions is a really effective mood lifter and can have a positive influence on our feelings of wellbeing.

These negative ions are created when air molecules are constantly being broken apart, for example by the rushing water of a waterfall or by the pounding of surf on a beach, and also by sunlight radiation and the energy, force and electricity in a lightning storm.

Next time a thunderstorm has blown through, remember to go outside and dose yourself in the energising effect of the newly purified air, breathe in and feel the calming effect of the negative ions.

Benjamin Franklin and the lightning rod. According to some, in June 1752, Benjamin Franklin built a kite with a sharp pointed wire attached to attract electrical charges (essentially a lightning rod). He attached, too, a key to the end of the kite string, near his holding hand, but held the kite with a silk ribbon that was tied to the key. **A thin metal wire**, also connected to the key, was inserted into a Leyden jar (a container for storing electrical charges). Then, during a thunderstorm, he let the kite fly. The kite was struck by lightning and cloud sparks (electrical charges/static electricity) travelled through the wet kite and string to the key and then into the Leyden jar. **Franklin noticed that loose fibres** on the string were bristling outwards because the string was charged with static electricity, so he intentionally reached out his knuckle to touch the key and he felt an electrical shock. The results of this experiment — the electrical shock to Franklin's hand, the charged Leyden jar and the string's bristling fibres — proved beyond any doubt that lightning is an electric phenomenon. Do not try this at home!

Star-gazing

Always remember we are under the same sky, looking at the same moon.
Maxine Lee

Shooting stars

When we look up into the inky night sky at the tiny twinkling lights and heavenly delights, we are looking far into the past, at stars that may no longer exist. It's a reminder that everything is temporary, it all passes, that we must remember to seize the moment, to try to do our best for the short time we are here.

Star-gazing is best done before the moon is full, as the moon creates its own bright light affecting what we see, and as far from urban areas as you can manage. In this part of Wales, we are in a dark sky area with minimal light pollution, away from the bright lights of towns or cities. Often, on a clear, dark, cloudless night we see stars and constellations in startling clarity. On such occasions, even the hazy, rippling band of the Milky Way takes on three dimensions, like a sponge of light, and it's possible to comprehend the size of the universe, to dream of infinity and beyond.

These magical streaks of light aren't actually stars but are caused by tiny bits of dust and rock called meteoroids falling into the Earth's atmosphere. The best way to see them is to lie flat on your back on a warm blanket and then to look up. Let your eyes relax and widen. Inevitably there'll be a shooting star when you are not looking. You need to be patient — and still. You can't rush these things. So relax and look straight up and allow the rod receptors at the periphery of the retina to become accustomed to the changes in light and dark, shape and movement. Once the rods catch the split second flash your eye will immediately turn to focus. I will admit, though, that I am completely hopeless at this, while James just looks up and sees them all the time, just as he always sees dolphins in the sea.

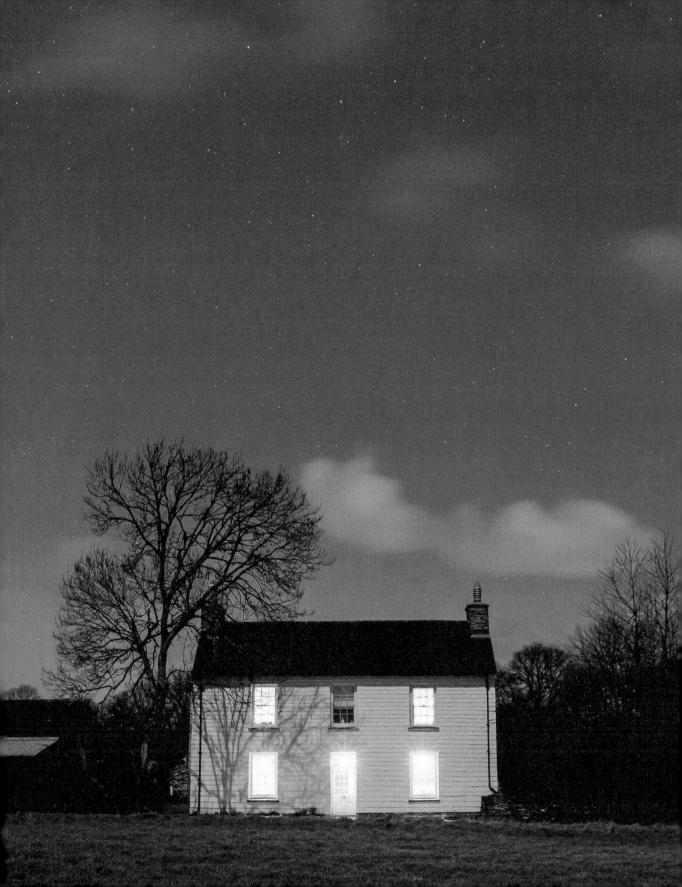

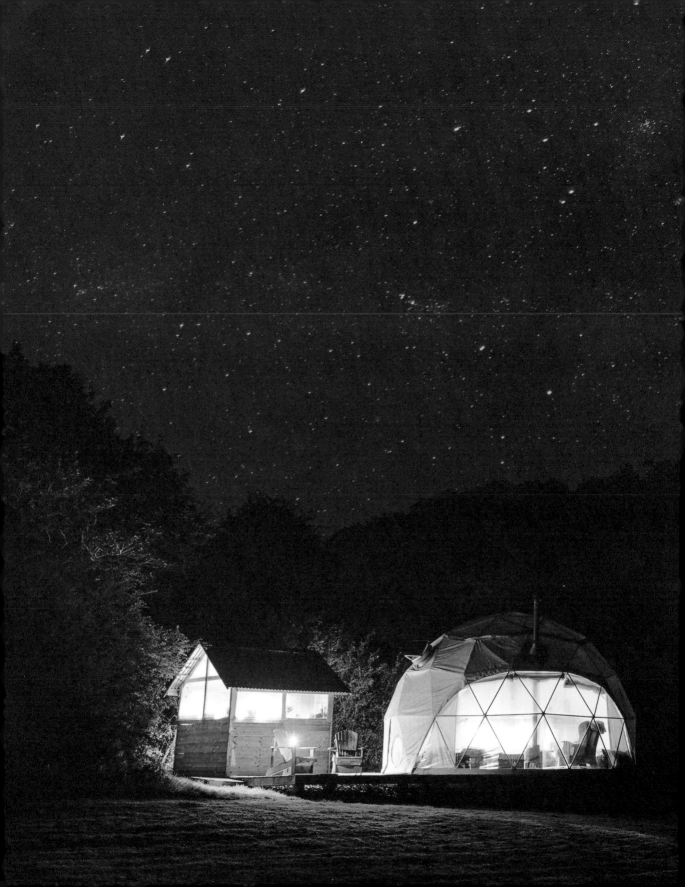

Changing seasons

Live in each season as it passes; breathe the air, drink the drink, taste the fruit, and resign yourself to the influence of the earth.
Henry David Thoreau

Each season has its own unique pleasures and advantages, but only by being outdoors can you truly appreciate these. A winter night is a living thing. It feels like an animal that wraps its arms around you, sapping your energy and sending you to sleep, into hibernation. By its end, I can't wait to see spring make its entrance. Each morning I look to see if the snowdrops have started to poke their heads out of the frozen earth, eager to see the flowers bloom and to hear the birds sing loudly again. In summer the longer days of sunlight encourage us to get up earlier and stay up later. Our bodies, like solar batteries, hold onto the sun's energy, helping us to gently power through the decline and fall of autumn.

At fforest we have learnt to trust in the change brought by the seasons, in the ebb and flow of life and the passing of time. Nothing stays the same, it is ever moving, growing and releasing.

Winter creeps in, slowing and cooling, bringing darkness. It is a greyer, gloomier time, with a colder, leafless landscape, stark of colour. It is a wonderful time to appreciate the form of trees, to see their majestic limbs and shape, their strong architectural structures, twigs peppered with lichen, moss and fern, a shine of evergreen. The long nights and short days allow time for rest and reflection, for cosying up by the fire, for recharging and planning for the new year ahead.

Spring brings cheer, excitement and new optimism. As nature awakens, the sap rises in the trees and bulbs, and buds emerge, bringing new growth and new beginnings.

Springtime slowly bursts with soft, pale yellow catkins, snowdrops, primroses, daffodils, zingy fresh new greens and delicate blossoms, wild garlic, wild anemone, blubells and hawthorn.

There is an explosion of birdsong and the emersion of animals, mating, nesting, hatching and hunting.

The sun shines warmer and brighter, the days grow longer, giving us the perfect opportunity to spend much more time outdoors.

Summer edges her way in, big and blowsy, full of warmth and lightness, bursting with enthusiasm, energy and abundance, all colours blooming and blazing.

It is a totally rich and vibrant time, luscious, bountiful and fruitful with harvest across the land and in the garden. The air is full with fragrance, bees and insects are buzzing and busy. We are at our busiest too, enjoying the warm, long days and endless magical summer evenings. We completely embrace the light, we stay up late and wake up early taking it all in.

Autumn brings generous harvests and rich warm glowing colours of burnished gold and ochre yellows, bronze, pumpkin, russets, roast chestnut, fox red, berry red and copper orange, which slowly seep through and then yield to bracken brown, earthy peaty smells of fungi, mushroom and damp leaves. It heralds the slow exhaustion of colour, a quietening of energy, a winding-down and total fall of foliage.

There is a cooler, softer, lower light, rainy and misty, moody and melancholy, as nature drifts into hibernation.

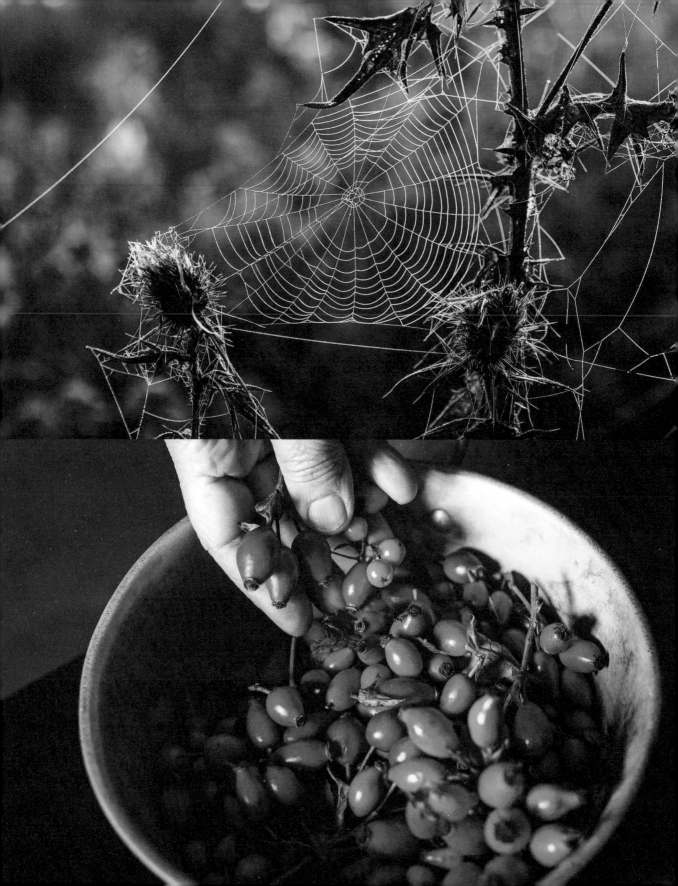

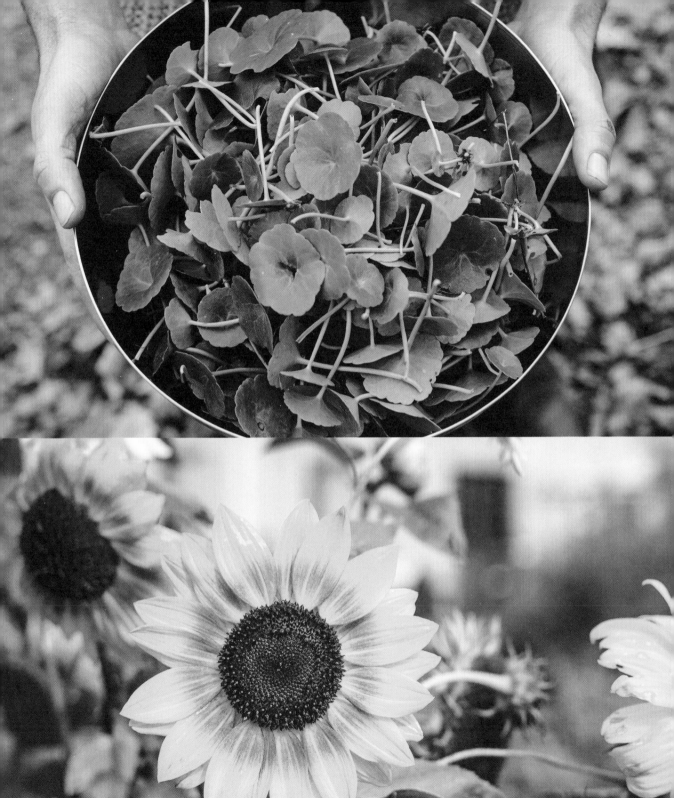

The beauty of birds

At fforest we leave large areas of land fallow, allowing nature the freedom to go wild, to turn back to scrub. This natural habitat, free from any agriculture, pesticides or sprays, encourages wild flowers and wild meadows, attracts bees and butterflies and also native birds, including buzzards, kites and peregrine falcons who can be seen circling their prey from above, as well as kingfishers and greater spotted woodpeckers.

It is hard to think of another natural occurrence or wonder that has quite such power to captivate and to stir our emotions as the annual cacophony of songs and calls that is the dawn chorus. No matter how cold, wet and grey the weather has been, all our winter blues are dispelled by this delightful sound of spring, so loud it rouses us from slumber yet still makes our hearts sing.

One of the earliest birds to start singing is the great tit and it's easy to distinguish its flinty notes (pee pee peep pee peep) ringing across the woods. By mid-spring the chorus reaches a crescendo, the happy chatter and squabble of sparrows mingling with the blackbird's ribbon of mellow song and the robin's bright and clear warbling. You might surprise yourself by how many of these songs you already know.

The sound of honking geese ushers in the autumn, as they fly in formation along the Teifi Gorge, all the way down the river to the sea and back, stretching and exercising their wings ready to fly south to warmer climes. From late autumn to winter, there are morning and evening murmurations of starlings flying to and fro over the reeds and wetlands to roost — a wonderful, compelling, natural phenomenon.

Feeding the birds

Encouraging birds into your garden is relatively easy. Tony, my dad, has always been passionate about feeding them, going out every morning to fill feeders with seeds and scraps of bread. As a result, he always has interesting birds to look at through the kitchen window while doing the washing up.

Tips for feeding the birds

Fat balls make excellent winter food. Birds need high-energy content to keep them warm. In the summer this need is reduced which is fortunate as fat balls tend to go soft and rancid in the sun.

Make your own bird cake balls by mixing melted suet or lard with seeds, nuts, dried fruit, oatmeal, cheese and cake. Use one-third fat to two-thirds other ingredients. Stir well, spoon into containers (empty coconut shells or plastic cartons make good feeders) and allow to set. Never use polyunsaturated margarines or vegetable oils for the fat as they can get smeared onto a bird's feathers, affecting their waterproofing and insulating qualities.

Dawn and dusk are the most important times of day to put out food, especially during colder months. In the summer, when they are moulting, birds still require high-protein food. There should be an abundance of insects and wild fruits, but a mix of black sunflower seeds, nuts, pinhead oatmeal, grated mild cheese and soaked dried fruits are all good to put out.

In summer keep feeders in the shade and make sure there is always a good fresh source of water.

Wild birds will only eat as much as they need so it isn't possible to over feed them.

Don't feed the birds junk food or kitchen waste.

If vermin and other pests become a problem, take away all the bird feeders. The birds will soon find other food sources and the pests will move on to forage in different places. After a week or two, you can put the feeders back out again and the birds will quickly return.

Never give birds milk as it can give them an upset stomach, or even cause death. They can, however, digest fermented dairy products, such as cheese. Grated mild cheese can be a good way of attracting robins or wrens.

Fresh coconut, straight from the shell, is good, but desiccated coconut can swell up in the stomachs of birds and cause death.

Bringing nature home

If you truly love nature,
you will find beauty everywhere.
Vincent van Gogh

First, let the sunshine in, roll up the blinds, pull back the curtains, open the windows and let in the natural light and fresh air. Unless it's howling a hoolie, freezing or pouring with rain, we will have the doors open too at fforest. Apart from the fresh air circulating and natural light coming in, views of natural things, like the sky and the trees, and the singing of a bird can have such a positive effect on our mood and attention.

James and I have a particular love for natural materials, especially wood, but also slate, stone and cloth. We know it is not to everybody's taste, but we find these natural elements are comforting, easy and reassuring. We feel the natural pattern and textures of these materials have an inherent quality of warmth and calm, making people feel relaxed and settled. Much of the wood, raw materials and furniture we use are either salvaged or recycled, and very often locally sourced. Our wool blankets are made, as they always were, in a mill not far away upstream from here.

Wild findings and foraged items brought home from walks and placed on a window sill or doorstep keep us connected to the outside. Pebbles, twigs, feathers, pieces of driftwood, shells, leaves and flowers are natural keepsakes. The little objects we pick up retain memories and carry stories of the people we were with and why we were there. They remind us of that time and space in nature, help us think clearly and recall a richness and calm.

fforest is littered with these treasures and natural arrangements. Wood stacked up under benches is there not only for practical reasons — to burn on the fire — but also because it is visually warming and pleasing, as are seasonal finds, such as flowers, seedheads and grasses, that are taken home to decorate the table.

For me, collecting natural things and then arranging them at home is both calming and therapeutic, almost a spiritual process, one that makes me feel happy and is utterly soothing. First, there is the gentle walk and wander outside, across a beach, on a woodland path, beside the riverbank or in the garden, along the way finding little treasures, picking them up, looking at them, admiring them and choosing the ones I'm going to take home with me. Throughout the year, there are always beautiful buds, flowers, seedheads, berries and foliage to be found, as well as pebbles, driftwood and sometimes shells too. Even lichen and moss-covered twigs in winter are a perfect simple decoration.

Then, when I get home, there is the arranging and rearranging, and the feeling of calm while faffing about in what might seem, to some, a pointless activity. I love to take time, looking at the colours and admiring the patterns of these organic, uneven objects and find joy in these simple things, at the space, balance and the harmony between each of them, and in making a pleasing arrangement. Enjoying these small moments of calm is, for me, a sort of meditation, a Zen-like moment. It mirrors the Japanese Shinto tradition where the Kami — sacred spirits found in the here and now of the natural world we live in — take the form of things and concepts important to life, such as the wind, rain, mountains, trees, wood, rivers, rocks and animals, and connect us back to nature.

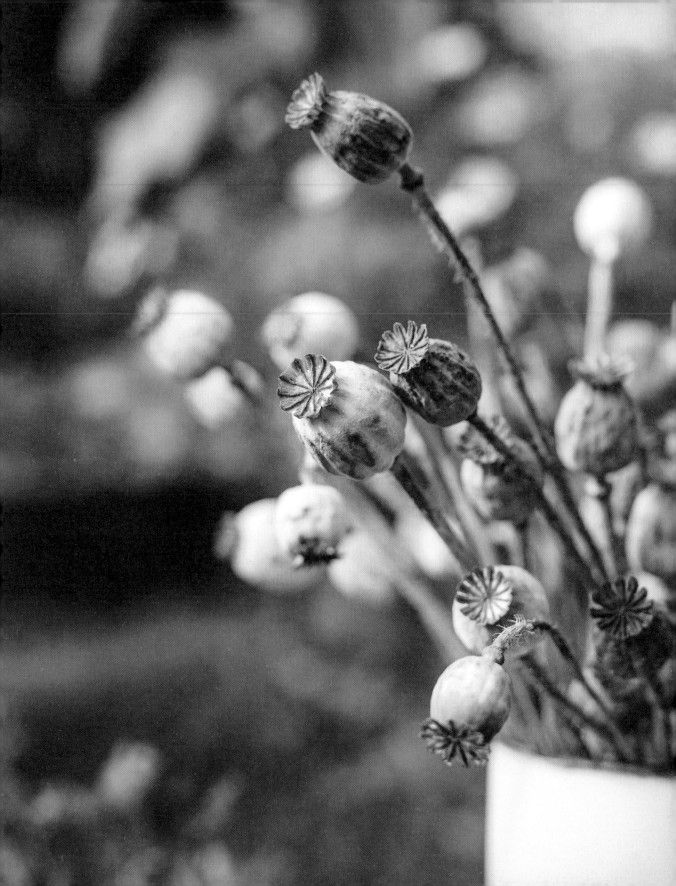

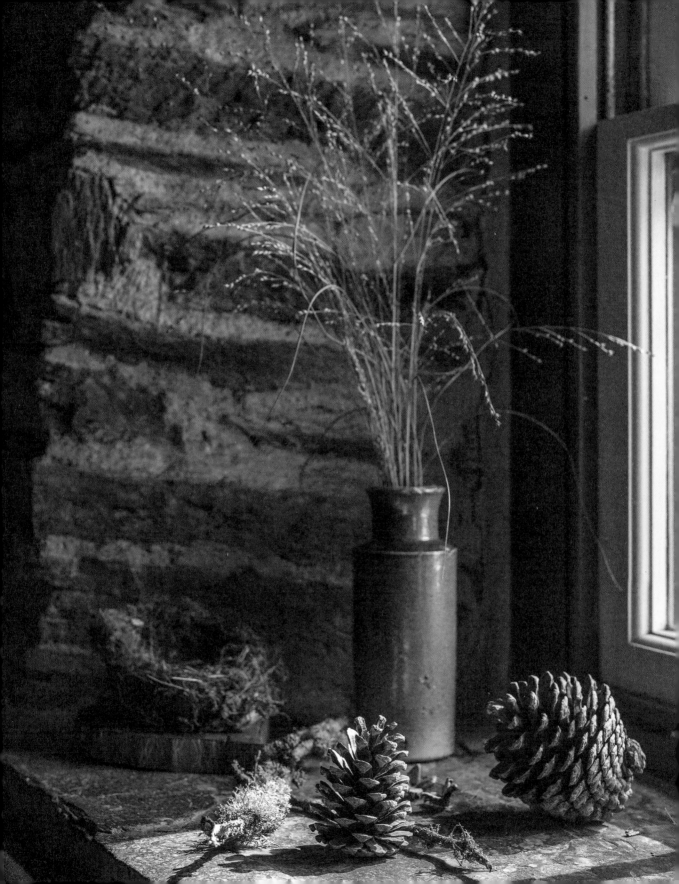

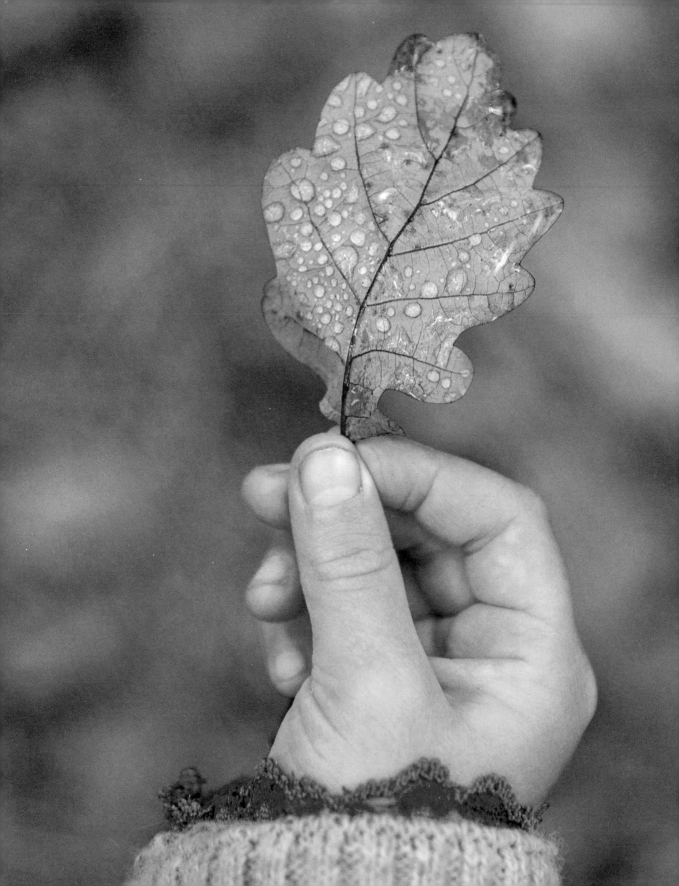

CREATING WITH NATURE

I go to nature to be soothed and healed,
and to have my senses put in order.
John Burroughs

Creativity happens in the absence of other things, often when you aren't doing anything in particular.

It can happen on a walk, in the shower, at your computer, on the phone, in the sea, fishing, or when you are asleep. When your mind can drift, it is free to grow and breathe and has time to ask questions.

We can look to nature for so much inspiration — for colour, design and pattern. Through studying the flexibility of a branch and how it bends, the structure of a feather or leaf, the symmetry of a snowflake, icicle or spider's web comes understanding. So many things have evolved, been designed and built as a result of looking to nature, from the principles of flight to the science of materials, including the use of natural dyes such as indigo, madder and onion skins.

At fforest we love to encourage the making of things and know that during the quiet time when our hands are busy doing tiny intricate projects our brain has time to be still, to drift and wonder, to be curious.

What follows in this chapter are some of the creative things we love to do and make.

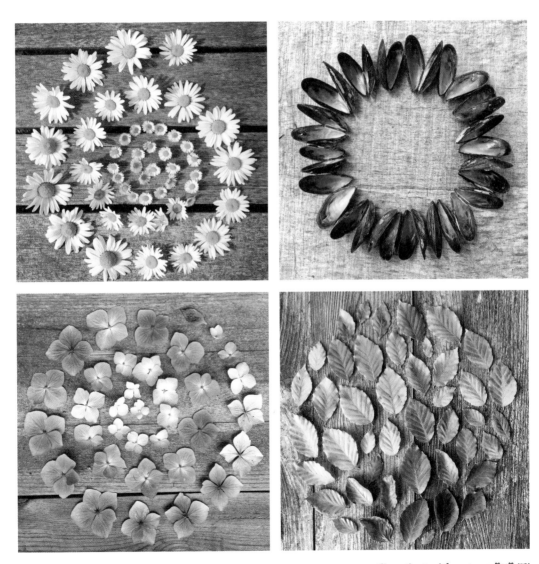

Collecting

I know a bank where the wild thyme blows,
Where oxlips and the nodding violet grows,
Quite over-canopied with luscious woodbine,
With sweet musk-roses and with eglantine.
A Midsummer Night's Dream, William Shakespeare

Why do we love flowers so much, what is their allure? Is it their colour, their symmetry and simplicity, the evocative scent, their delicacy and fragility, the fact that they symbolise love, or the connection they make with our ancestors who also foraged for food and flowers? We love them for all these reasons, and because they always evoke happiness and delight.

From the very beginning of fforest, one thing was very clear to me, we would always have freshly picked wild flowers. Seasonal posies offer a wonderful welcome, they bring a gentle connection to the land and add a real sense of season, time and place.

When I wander out to the fields, shoreline and woods to forage and collect there is an ever-changing palette of colours, textures and patterns to choose from. I pick only the flowers and vegetation that are available in the garden or grow wild. The fragile beauty of many of these wild flowers means they would never survive commercial processing, so they have an 'extra special' element that is difficult to achieve with bought flowers.

Flowers always make people better, happier, and more helpful; they are sunshine, food and medicine to the mind.
Luther Burbank

Below are a few things you really must take into consideration when you go out to collect things.

Always be mindful of laws on trespassing.

Do not forage on protected sites. Unless you are on common land, open access land or a public right of way, you are trespassing by entering land without the owner's permission.

Always be respectful of preserving a biodiverse and sustainable environment.

Only collect flowers, leaves, fruits and seeds where they are plentiful, making sure there is enough left for the birds and wildlife.

In the UK it is not an offence to take away foliage, fruit or parts of the plant that are growing wild, if you are not taking them for commercial purposes, but elsewhere it's important to check local regulations.

Never take away the whole plant or its roots. Always take care to avoid damage to the plant and the roots so that it can continue to grow naturally and flourish.

It is always wise to avoid areas of pollution, where crops have been sprayed and alongside busy roads.

Mid-winter snowdrops, ferns, hazel catkins.
Late winter nettles emerging, sweet violets, dandelions, willow catkins, pussywillows, camellias, hellebores, blackthorn blossoms. **Early spring** gorse flowers, daffodils, cleavers, wild garlic, hawthorn leaves, primroses, red campion, marsh marigolds, wood anemones, periwinkles, euphorbias, magnolias. **Mid-spring** cow parsley, jack-in-the-hedge, young bramble leaves, hairy bittercress, tulips, bluebells, stitchwort, forget-me-not, lady's mantel, dog violets, cherry blossom, cowslip. **Late spring** hawthorn flower, ox-eye daisies, red clover, sorrel, hogweed, watercress, foxgloves, thrift, cowslips, comfrey, oak blossom, lilac. **Early summer** mallow, honeysuckle, roses, elderflowers, chamomile, welsh poppies, common poppies, ground elder, meadow crane's-bill, corn flowers, irises, alliums, borage, grasses, daisies. **Mid-summer** strawberries, yarrow, meadow sweet, horseradish, sweet cicely, rosebay willowherb, fennel, nasturtiums, thistles, nigella, sweetpeas, purple tufted vetch, wild carrot. **Late summer** blackberries begin, rowan berries, wild carrots, marigolds, lavender, sunflowers, mint and sage flowers, yarrow, coriander seeds. **Early autumn** beechnuts, crab apples, elderberries, haws, damsons, hazelnuts, rosehips, walnuts, apples, pears, acorns, ferns, hydrangers, wild carrot seedheads. **Mid-autumn** sloes, sweet chestnuts, conkers, burdock, crabapples, seedheads, hawthorn berries. **Late autumn** pine cones, teazles, Chinese lanterns. **Early winter** pennywort, holly, ivy, lichens, pine, twigs.

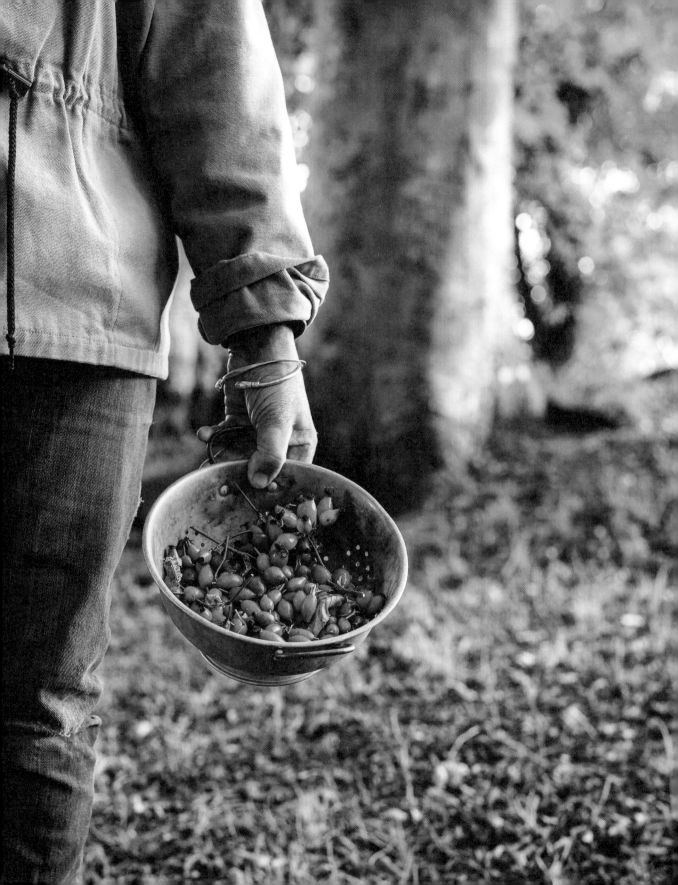

Pressing flowers and leaves

Pressing flowers, weighting them flat as they dry, has been done for centuries, since as long ago as Ancient Egyptian times. It's a technique that allows us not only to preserve the flowers' delicate beauty but also the memories we associate with them. The Japanese art of oshibana, which uses pressed flowers, petals and leaves to create elaborate images, dates back to the 1500s, but only became known in the West when trade increased between Japan and Europe in the late 1890s. It then became very fashionable in Victorian England. It requires meticulous skill and is said to have been an art perfected by samurai warriors to promote patience and harmony with nature.

It's not merely a decorative pastime, however. The examples found in scrapbooks of plants and flowers collected and pressed by travellers, gardeners and botanists have also improved our knowledge of nature and the botanical world.

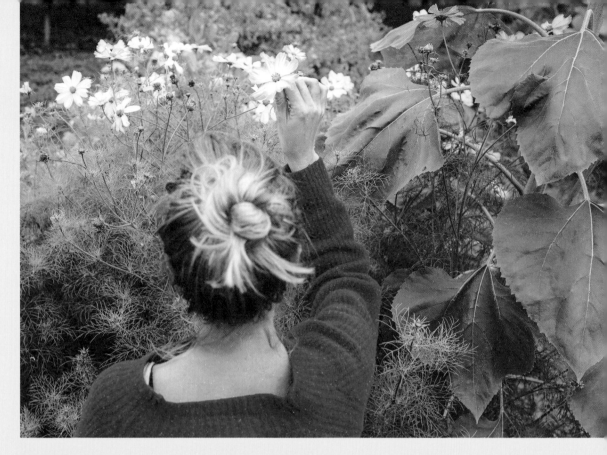

Method

To retain maximum colour and prevent browning, flowers have to be fresh but dry, so choose ones that are either in bud or have just blossomed, and pick them on a sunny day.

Begin with a small, flat flower, such as a daisy, primrose or pansy. Large, bulky flowers will need trimming at the back to get them to lay flat.

Use either a special flower press, which can be bought easily in shops or online, or heavy books, such as big dictionaries, an encyclopaedia or even old telephone books.

Moisture from the flowers may cause the pages to wrinkle a bit, so avoid using a book you don't want damaged. To help prevent this, put the flower(s) between two pieces of paper before placing them between the pages of the book. Printer paper, blotting paper, thin cardboard, plain non-treated tissue and even coffee filters can be used. It is best, however, to avoid kitchen paper and patterned papers as many have textures and colour that may end up imprinted on the petals.

Arrange the flat face of the flower on your paper, then press it within the pages of the book.

You can press multiple flowers at the same time, just ensure there is sufficient space between them so that moisture from one flower doesn't transfer and they don't become stuck to one another.

Do not disturb the arrangement when closing the book. Use more books, or a brick, to weigh down the book once it is closed. Leave for at least a couple of weeks until the flowers have dried out.

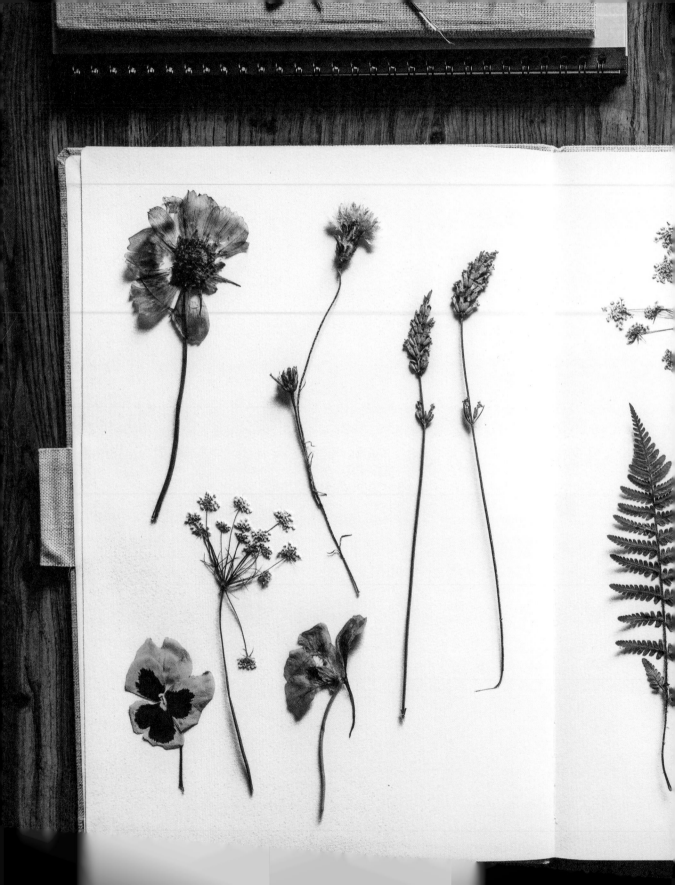

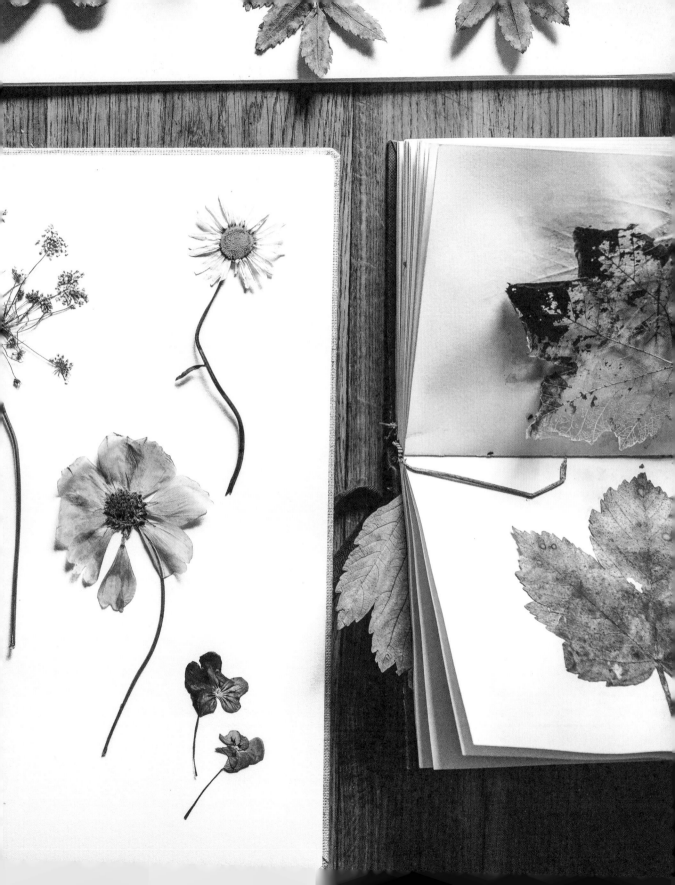

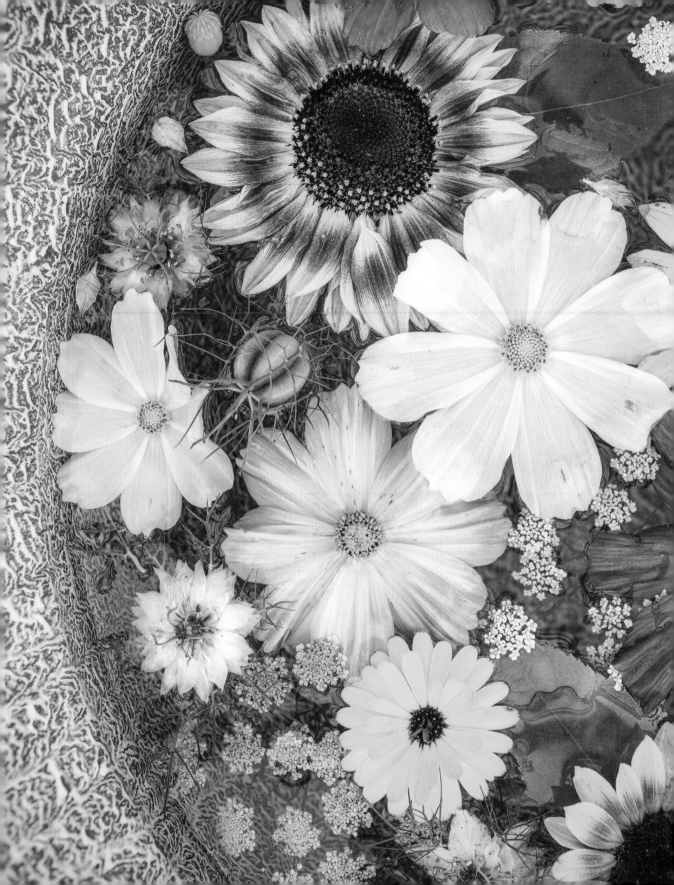

Floating flowers

Water, thou hast no taste, no colour, no odour;
canst not be defined, art relished while ever
mysterious. Not necessary to life, but rather
life itself.
Antoine de Saint-Exupéry

Having nature inside and outside our home brings beauty and a wonderful sense of peace and tranquility. Flowers within the home add grace and pleasure and cheer up our emotions enormously. The sight, sound and smell can all produce a mood of peacefulness and harmony.

When I was younger, I travelled in India and noticed that instead of putting flowers in vases as a welcome it was common to find bowls or pools of water filled with floating flowers and foliage. I have loved this way of bringing nature into the home ever since.

The practice is rooted in the ancient Hindu principles of Vastu, which focus on the natural environment and the five elements and energies of nature: earth, space, water, fire and air. Maintaining a positive balance with our environment encourages good energy, harmony and flow, crucial to health, peace and happiness.

Water, as rain, rivers and the seas, is precious and holds great energy. It is the essence of life, the basis of all life; without water, life cannot exist. Placing a bowl filled with water and flowers near the entrance to your home is therefore highly auspicious.

Method

Take a bowl, I prefer a shallow, wide bowl, and fill it with cold water.

Cut the stems of the flowers about 3–5 cm (1–2in) long so they can still suck up the water to keep hydrated. Flat flowers with a larger surface area will float best.

Float your freshly picked leaves and flowers on top of the water — like lily pads — to create your own delightful floral pond.

A seashell wind chime

The shore is an ancient world, for as long as there has been an earth and sea there has been this place of the meeting of land and water.
Rachel Carson

Almost every day I go to the beach, and pretty much always come back with something from the shoreline. In particular sea shells — I love their seemingly delicate but solid structure, and their incredible patterns and colours. I look at them and wonder what has lived in them, how they were made.

I have so many shells, as well as pebbles, pieces of sea glass and driftwood, that they are displayed on window ledges, in flowerpots, on the ground and on the wall.

A wonderful thing to have and make with your finds is a wind chime, to hang indoors, in the bathroom window, the porch or outside on a branch of a tree — anywhere that feels perfect to you and makes you happy.

Wherever you put this, it will always remind you of the sea.

You will need

seashells. If you like, you can also use sea glass, maybe beads or buttons, feathers and leaves, whatever you have or takes your fancy

some fishing line or twine, thin string or strong thread

a drill and a small drill bit if you need to make some holes in the shells, although I like to find shells that already have a little worn hole in them

a biggish piece of driftwood from which to hang the strings of shells

Method

Hold each shell between your finger and thumb and dip it in freshwater to clean away any sand or dirt. Take the time to admire your shells and think about the design you are going to make.

Take a length of twine and thread it through each shell, tying each one securely so it doesn't slip down onto the shell below, unless that is the look you want to achieve. If necessary, use a drill fitted with a small drill bit to make holes in the shells.

Add each shell, one by one, until you have as many as you want on each length of twine.

Tie each of your strings of shells securely to your piece of driftwood. When you have the right effect, you can tie some twine to the top of the driftwood in order to hang it up.

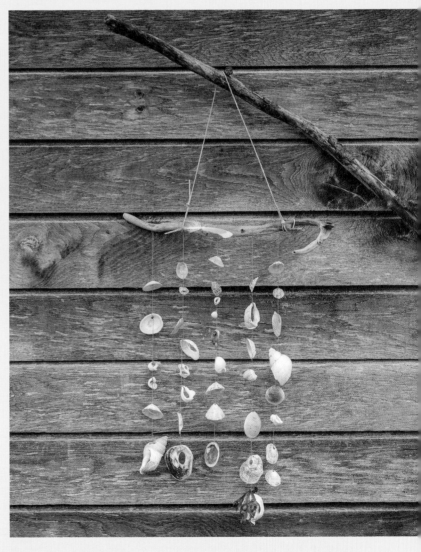

A seasonal wreath

Making a wreath gets you a little closer to nature and is a wonderful way to celebrate seasonal changes and bring indoors a little bit of feelgood wildness.

You can do this any time of the year, not just at Christmas. Spring, summer, autumn or winter, there is always something interesting to find, including leafy twigs, lichen- or moss-covered twigs, freshly sprouting buds and catkins, ivy, dried seedheads, honesty, grasses, old man's beard, rosehips, teasels, lavender, bayleaves and cow parsley. When out on a walk take a few cuttings; it is always handy to have secateurs in your bag to collect things that catch your eye.

Really have some fun and get creative. There are no rules about doing this, and there is no need to cover the whole wreath base if you don't want to. Some people like to make a wreath with perfect symmetry, while others prefer a more quirky, chaotic and untamed wildness.

You will need

secateurs or floristry scissors

willow to make your own wreath or a pre-made wreath base, which is a great investment as you can use it again and again

ribbon or twine to hang the wreath

some twine or floristry wire to tie things in

your collected finds — dried flowers, fresh flowers, foliage, seedheads, the more natural and wilder the better

Things to consider

Look for different textures, colour balance, a variety of shapes of flowers and leaves.

Fresh flowers in the wreath are not kept in water so will not last long (though it will depend on the flower). It is best to add these at the last minute if making the wreath for a special occasion.

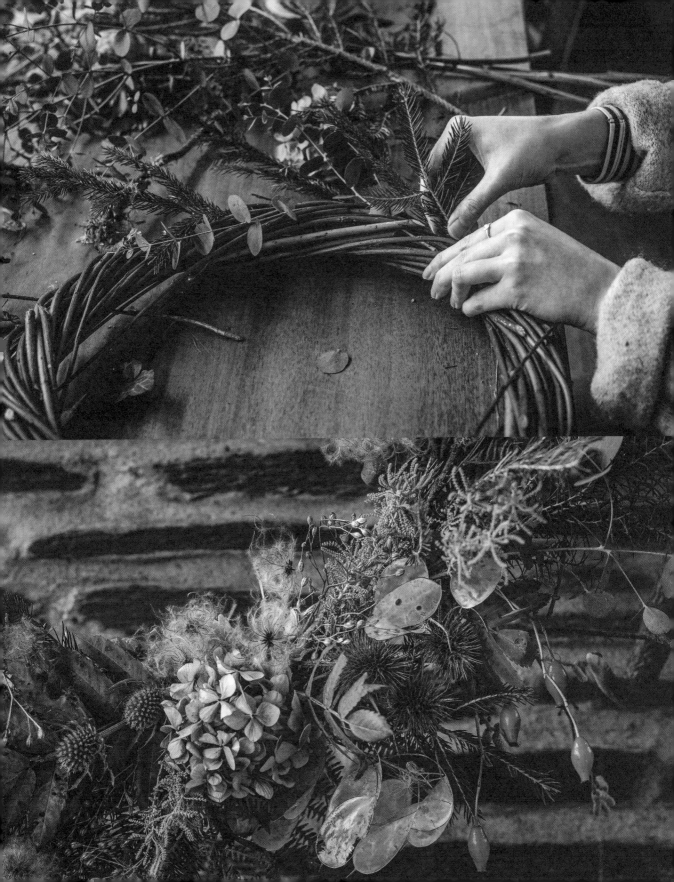

A long exposure photo of the night sky

Here are some tips on how to capture the wonders and magnificence of the sky at night from Finn, the photographer who took the beautiful pictures in this book.

Tips for photographing the night sky

Dark skies are crucial. Any artificial light from towns or streetlights will pollute the sky and dim the light from the stars, so it's best to head into the countryside. There are a number of dark sky preserves in the UK, which are areas that restrict artificial light pollution to promote astronomy. Even the moon can contribute to light pollution, a full moon or even a half moon is really bright so choose a night when the moon is in its first lunar phase: the new moon.

Watch the weather. Cloud cover is an obvious deterrent to star photography, but remember, too, that wind is a nightmare for long exposures!

I prefer to shoot the night sky with some foreground interest — something on the ground to set the sky against — I think it provides some perspective to the enormity of the night sky. Plan in the daytime where you are going to shoot and scout for any hazards you might not see in the dark.

Remember it might be cold and you will probably be out for quite some time, so make sure you wrap up warm or at least take another layer; "you can always take a layer off, but you can't put one on" as my mother used to say!

You will need a sturdy, well-built tripod and, ideally, a cable release to eliminate camera shake — some exposures may be up to 25 seconds long. If you don't have a cable release, use your camera's self-timer instead. A 2-second delay is all you need to press the button and move your hand away so that you're not touching the camera (and causing vibration).

A fast, wide-angle lens that has a manual focus setting is key since your autofocus will not work at night. Adjust your lens to focus at infinity, or at a faraway horizon. Experiment with different ISOs and aperture settings, and above all enjoy the experience of being underneath the most mind-boggling ceiling you will ever see.

Printing with the sun

Sun printing, also known as cyanotype, or 'blueprinting', is a wonderful way to capture the summer sunshine and make botanical prints of your favourite flowers, leaves, seeds and foliage.

Using sunlight or UV light to develop a chemically treated paper is the oldest photographic printing process. It was invented in 1842 by Sir John Herschel and later refined by botanist Anna Atkins who used the light-sensitive paper to reproduce simple one-colour images of her favourite plant specimens to make cyanotype books documenting her botanical finds. As a result, she is regarded as the first female photographer.

A local photographer, friend and contributor to events at fforest, Kate Dunwell, taught us how to print with the sun and this is the way we do it.

Method

Prepare the paper. It doesn't matter what kind of watercolour paper you use, as long as it's uncoated. You don't want any chemicals in the paper to mix with the chemicals you're using for the cyanotype process.

Make the solution. Pre-mix and dissolve separately each of the two chemicals listed below in 100ml (3½ fl oz) of distilled water. Both chemicals, which are readily available online, are iron salts. When exposed to ultraviolet light they are reduced to their ferrous state, producing a high contrast blue image.

25g (1oz) ferric ammonium citrate (green).

10g (¼ oz) potassium ferricyanide.

Store these solutions separately until needed.

When you want to print, make the active solution by mixing equal quantities of both solutions. Do this very carefully; you don't want it to spill as stains won't come out. The shelf life of this solution is a lot shorter than that of the two separate ones.

Paint or sponge the solution evenly onto the paper in a room with no sunlight at all. The process is sensitive to UV light only, so at night, after dark, it's perfectly safe to have the lights on. There's no need for safe lights.

After coating, let the paper dry for at least 24 hours in a really dark place with no daylight. An airing cupboard is good. When the paper is dry, keep it in a black 'light proof' bag so it doesn't get exposed to any light at all before you need it.

Negative or positive images are made by blocking UV light from reaching the sensitised paper to create the picture. To do this, place a leaf, flower, seaweed, paper-cut design or whatever you want on the prepared paper and expose it to sunlight for 10–15 minutes, depending how strong the sun is. If you place a piece of glass over the top while you are exposing, this stops the leaf blowing away and helps to keep a sharper edge.

Rinse the paper in a bath of cold tap water for at least 30 seconds to completely wash off all the solution. The print will keep on developing for some time during and after washing, so don't worry if your pattern looks as if it is disappearing. The paper will retain the image of the leaf after it has been rinsed.

Hang the paper up to dry in the wind and the sunshine. The areas that were exposed to the sun will turn from a muddy green to a beautiful shade of Prussian blue. Those that were covered by the leaf will stay paper-white.

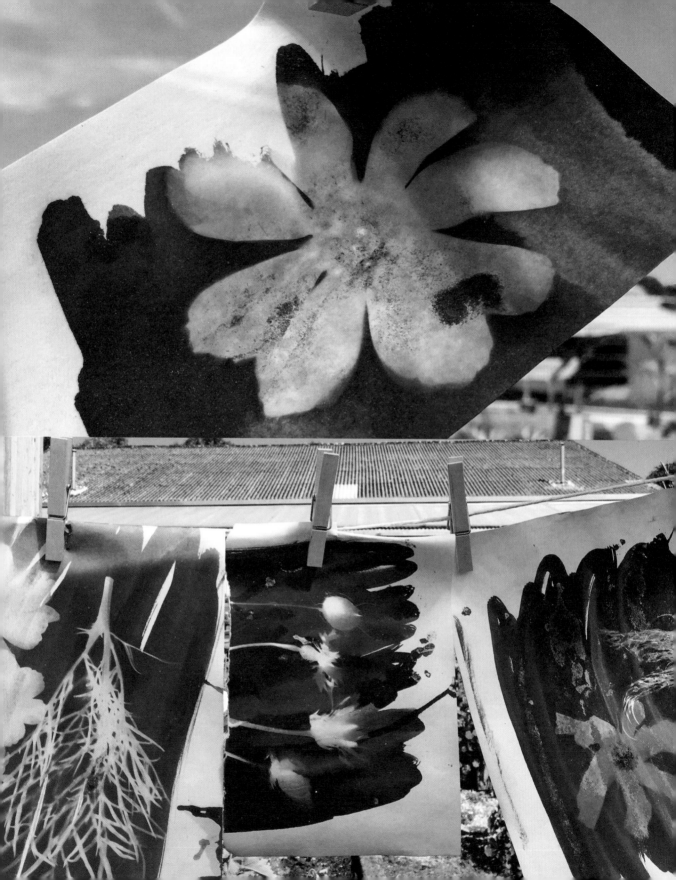

Growing

The glory of gardening: hands in the dirt,
head in the sun, heart with nature. To nurture
a garden is to feed not just the body, but the soul.
Alfred Austin

The joy of gardening begins in winter, before it is possible to plant anything. There is pleasure and satisfaction to be had in planning and deciding what exactly you are going to grow. We get our seeds from Real Seeds, a small farm in Pembrokeshire, that supplies seeds from old heirloom varieties.

In spring, there is the joy of being outside, feeling your arms and legs warm up, digging, weeding and nurturing your seedlings, watching them sprout and grow while listening to the birds sing, observing the bees buzz and the butterflies flutter doing their important job of pollinating. We often see little frogs amongst the plants searching for slugs and bugs to eat, and the amazing pale copper brown, smooth, metallic and shiny slowworms that live in the polytunnel too; their favourite food is the bugs that eat the greens.

If this sounds all a bit too bucolic, let's not forget the weather: cold Baltic winds and freezing fingers, grey pouring rain and soggy dripping bobble hats, runny noses and damp squelchy boots, even when it's hot, and it's too hot sometimes!

But this is offset by the rewarding and blissful moment when you go out amongst the plants and spot the first red tomato, find the first juicy strawberry or when you pick the first of the season's vegetables. When we harvest and gather our own food the brain releases the 'happy chemical' dopamine. A sense of wellbeing and elation can be can be triggered just by seeing the fruit or berry, by its scent, as well as the action of actually picking it. These reactions are buried deep in our DNA, from our hunter-gather ancestors.

Serotonin, another happy chemical, is likewise triggered through activity and achievement, such as when we are in the garden getting our hands dirty. Mycobacterium vaccae, a bacteria found in good healthy soil, also triggers the release of serotonin.

From the beginning of fforest, growing our own food and flowers was always high up on the list as being very important to us. The first year for us was a haze of fast learning. Creating a warm and interesting space was the easy part. Even though we always loved to have friends to stay, learning about the 'business' of hospitality, welcoming and looking after people, involved a lot of adjustment.

In August 2007, the first year of fforest being open, a young couple turned up one afternoon at the Lodge door holding baskets of homegrown vegetables they wanted us to buy. They were dressed in matching stripy Breton tops and wore huge smiles. That is when we met Alice Holden.

Not long afterwards, work on the fforest produce garden began. Alice pretty much built the raised beds and put up the polytunnel all on her own. She dug up a gazillion long stubborn dock roots, dug tons of compost into the beds and planted our first garden. For this we are forever grateful.

Alice established a wonderfully productive vegetable patch — and set us on our way on keeping healthy compost. After Alice, Tamsin took over the garden fork and continued the growing. Now it is Brook and Danny who keep the garden beautiful and us all delighted and nourished with great produce. It's interesting to note that all our gardeners have been women.

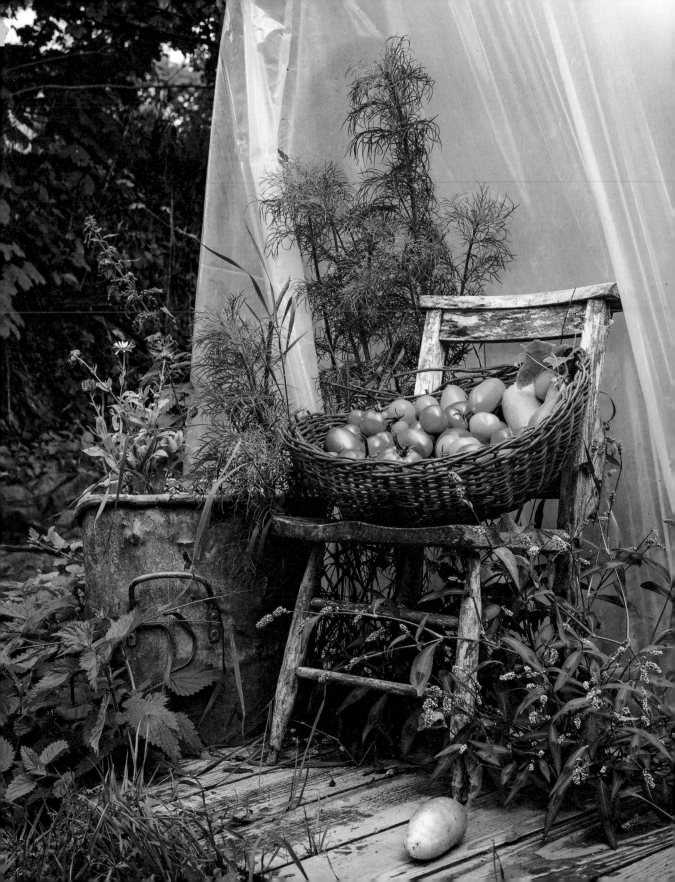

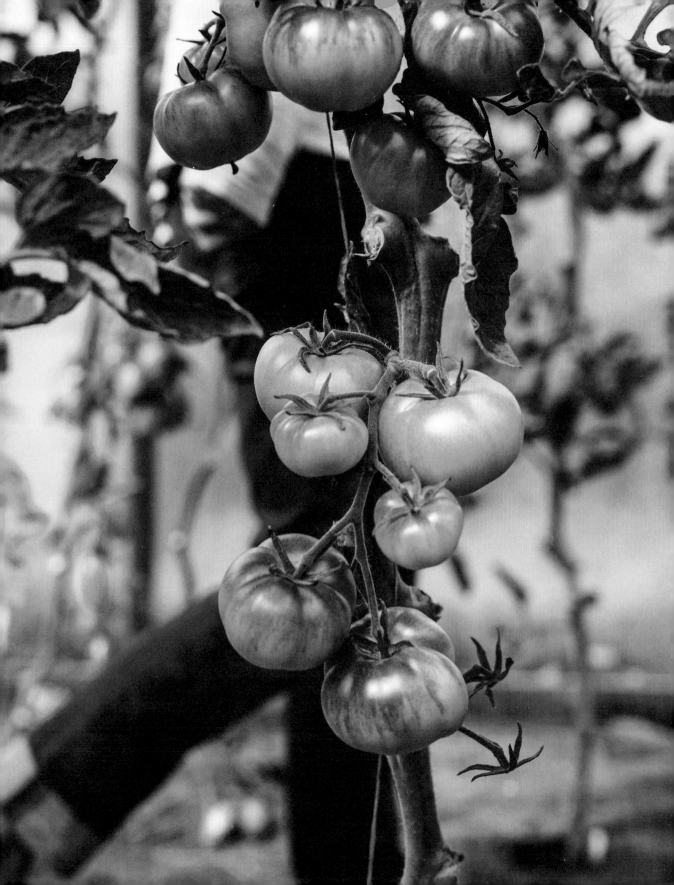

Compost

Making good compost is an essential part of maintaining a healthy and fruitful garden. The tips below come from Brook, our gardener at fforest.

Tips for composting

Old pallets make perfect compost bins. Four around the sides and none on the bottom will give plenty of aeration to the pile and provide easy access for the worms. We cover our compost with a tarp to keep in the moisture. If you don't fancy building a compost heap, or you don't have the know-how, there are plenty of good ones available to buy.

Find the perfect position. A sunny spot is good, the warmth helps to break down everything quickly, and a level and well-drained position is best, somewhere any excess water will drain away easily. You don't want it getting waterlogged or going mouldy. Ideally you want worms to move in and munch up and break down all the matter.

What to compost All the green stuff, such as raw vegetable peelings and fruit waste, but also coffee grounds, teabags, grass cuttings (though too much creates excess nitrogen), egg shells, plant prunings and plant trimmings. If you can get seaweed, this is also very good. All these break down quickly, providing moisture and nitrogen to the mix.

Scrunched up newspaper, cardboard, wood chippings, paper napkins and fallen autumn leaves —, what we call the brown stuff is slower to rot but add vital fibre and carbon to your compost. It also creates essential air pockets in the mixture.

Never add any diseased plants, perennial weeds such as bindweed, dock roots, ragwort, thistle or weeds with seedheads. (You want to avoid these plants popping up and growing amongst your much wanted ones.) Never ever put any cooked foods, meat or dairy products, nappies, cat or dog poo in the compost, otherwise it will begin to stink and will lead to unwanted flies and pests.

The key to good compost lies in getting a good balance and the right mix of 'greens' and 'browns'. Ideally it is best to have 30:1 brown to green.

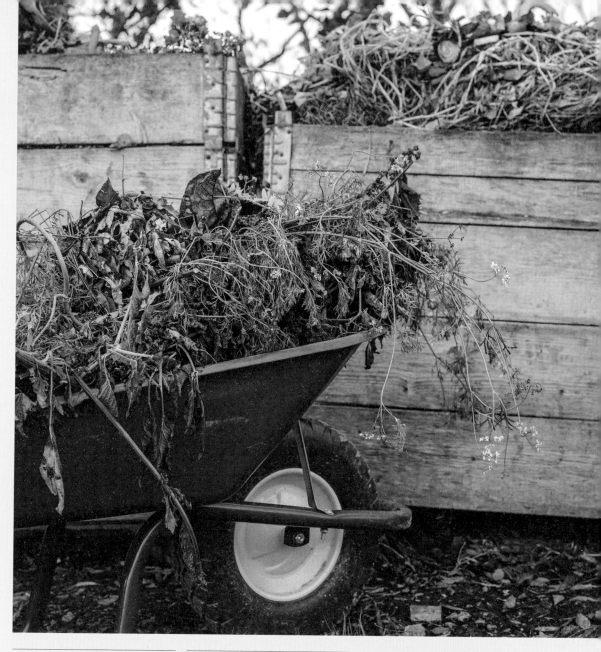

If your compost is too wet, add more of the brown stuff.

If it's too dry, add some more of the green stuff.

Turning your compost regularly helps to aerate and mix up the waste and aids faster composting.

It's ready when you have a dark brown, almost black healthy hummus, it should have a spongy texture and smell good. Spreading this compost on your beds to a depth of about 5cm (2in) every autumn and spring will greatly improve your soil quality and help you grow healthy, beautiful blooms and bountiful harvests, free from sprays and chemical fertilisers.

Spring wild leaf pesto

A tonic for the spring made from nettles and wild garlic.

So much super-healthy natural goodness is found in the tender, silky wild garlic leaves and early, earthy nettles. Wild garlic is full of vitamins A and C, which are potent antioxidants, as well as calcium, potassium, magnesium and iron.

Nettles are also high in iron and vitamin C and are an ideal detoxifier. Raw wild garlic can be pretty overpowering, but nettles are a perfect partner to calm it down.

Please wear gloves when you go out to pick the nettles, since young fresh nettle tops really do sting, as I can vouch for! My fingers tingled for two days after picking nettles without protecting my hands. If you do get stung, find some dock leaves to rub into the affected area. It might well be an old wives' tale, but it always seems to work for me.

Ingredients

40g (1½ oz) fresh wild garlic leaves

40g (1½ oz) fresh young nettle tips (top 2–6 leaves), picked before flowering

juice of 1 lemon

4–5 tablespoons olive oil

40–60g (1½–2¼ oz) nuts, such as pine nuts, cashews, hazelnuts, pecans, walnuts, whatever you fancy

30g (1oz) Parmesan or similarly strong, hard cheese, finely grated

sea salt

freshly ground black pepper

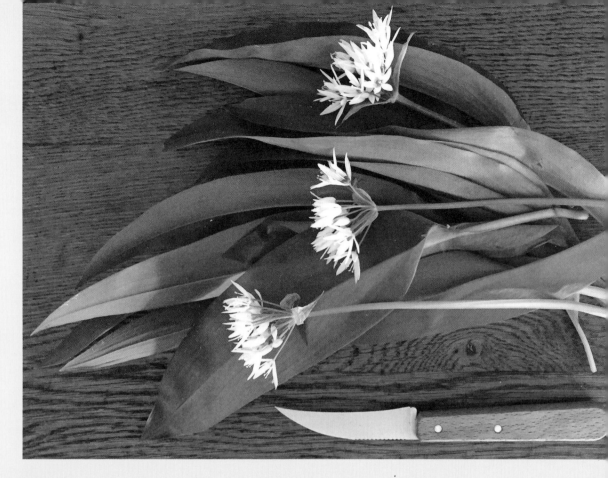

Method

Wash the wild garlic leaves well, then wash the nettle leaves well (remember to wear gloves). Steam or blanch the nettle leaves for a minute or two, to remove the sting. Once cooled, squeeze out the excess water and chop roughly.

Whizz all the leaves in a blender with half the lemon juice and enough of the olive oil to loosen the mix.

Dry roast the nuts in a frying pan till golden brown.

Add the nuts to the blender and process until smooth or the pesto is to a consistency of your liking.

Spoon into a bowl and stir in the cheese. Stir in more olive oil as needed and the remainder of the lemon juice. Season with salt and pepper.

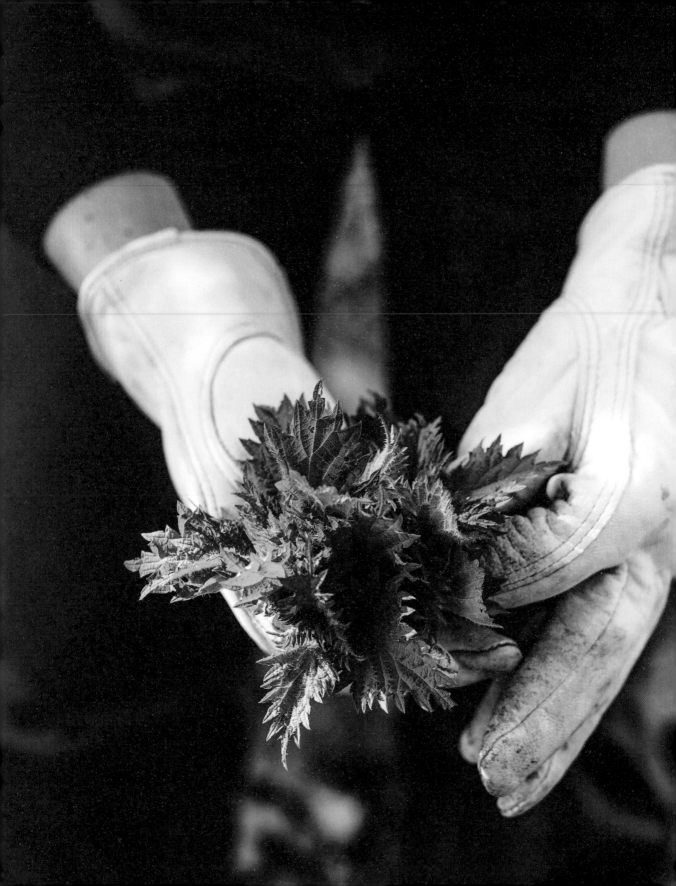

Spring nettle cake

A life-enhancing cake for early spring.

This cake is a gorgeous fresh green colour and, because of the lemon and sugar, it doesn't taste savoury, the irony rich umami flavour of the nettles giving way to citrus.

When you get your young nettle tops back to the kitchen, carefully wash them, removing the stems before quickly blanching in a pan of boiling water for a couple of minutes to remove the sting. Do not cook for too long or the nettles will lose their bright green colour and become a dull khaki. Drain and refresh immediately in ice-cold water to stop the cooking. Drain, then blitz in a food processor.

Ingredients

200g (7oz) unsalted butter, at room temperature

150g (5½ oz) caster sugar

6 eggs

2 teaspoons vanilla extract

4 tablespoons lemon juice

zest of 1 lemon

100g (3½ oz) nettles, prepared as above

250g (9oz) plain flour, plus extra for dusting

2 teaspoons baking powder

pinch of salt

Method

Preheat the oven to 170°C (325°F), Gas Mark 3. Baking at this lower temperature helps the cake to retain its fresh green colour.

Lightly grease and flour two 18cm (7in) cake tins. Cut out a circle of parchment paper to fit the bottom and grease and flour this too.

In a large bowl, cream the butter and sugar. Beat in the eggs, one at a time, until they are well combined.

Beat in the nettle purée. Add the vanilla, lemon juice and zest and mix well. Sift in the flour, baking powder, and salt. Mix well.

Pour into the prepared cake tins and bake for about 25 minutes or until a skewer inserted in the centre comes out clean. Rest for a while in the tins before turning out onto a wire rack to cool.

To serve the cake, drizzle with icing or layer and cover with a creamy lemon butter icing made by creaming 150g softened unsalted butter, then beating in 300g icing sugar and the zest and juice of ½ a lemon until nice and smooth.

Decorate with sugared primroses on page 86.

Sugaring flowers

Sugared flowers are oh so pretty and so very satisfying when used to decorate your cakes. All you need are petals from edible flowers, egg white and sugar.

The most commonly used flowers are: roses, violets, primroses, pansies, cherry blossom, nasturtiums, marigolds, borage carnations, dandelions, red clover, honeysuckle and lilacs.

Tips for making sugared flowers

Always make sure your flowers are clean and dry before you begin. You can use individual petals separated from the flower, or whole small flowers, such as violets, blossom, borage and primroses.

Use the white of one egg to 50g (1¾oz) of sugar. Icing sugar gives a subtle, matte appearance. Use caster sugar if you'd like a crystallised, sugary look.

Paint the petals or the flowers all over with egg white or gently dip them into egg white.

Then sprinkle with or dip into sugar, which will stick to the egg white.

Dry overnight on greaseproof paper in a warm and dry place. And enjoy the happiness of decorating.

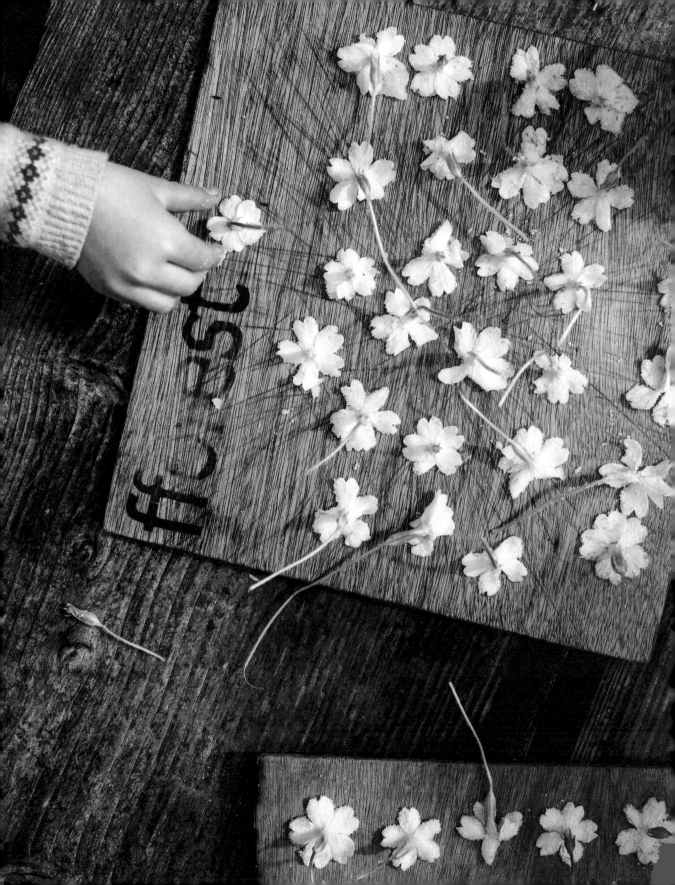

Herbal teas

The benefits of herbal teas have been recognised for thousands of years. Apart from being refreshing and tasty to drink, many herbs have health-giving minerals and properties, helping to detoxify and even strengthen our immune system.

I came to tea quite late in life and herbal tea even later, never really liking the dried leaves and flowers out of a packet, as they always tasted a bit bitter to me. It was only when I was given tea made with fresh mint leaves or slices of fresh ginger that I began to love and appreciate the refreshing, clean taste.

Whenever possible, and it is always the loveliest way, pick the herbs as you need them to make your tea. If you don't have a garden you can grow them in a plant pot on your window sill. Just a few leaves or flowers per person in the teapot is enough. Pour freshly boiled water onto them and leave to brew for a few minutes before drinking. Alternatively, and this is what I prefer to do, put your herbs in a cup or in a strong glass so you can see the gorgeous colour and shape of the flowers and leaves while drinking. My particular favourites are dandelion, nettle, elderflower, mint, fennel and pine needle.

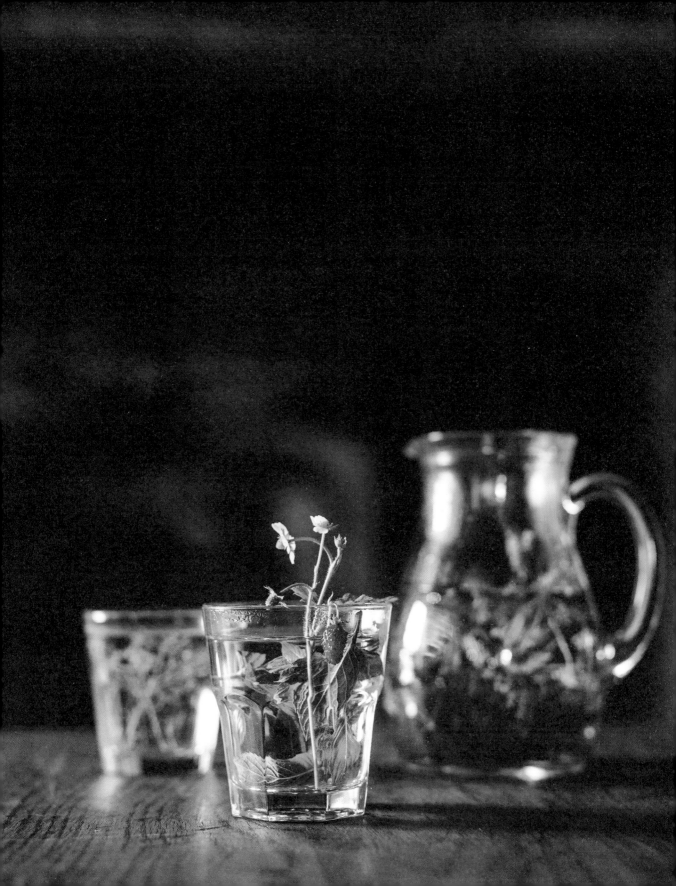

Summer herbal healing balm

A beautifully simple way of capturing the radiance of summer-flowering herbs.

This way of naturally nurturing your skin comes from our dear friend Reidin, of Warrior Botanicals, who came all the way from Ireland to share her recipes with us.

Ingredients

1 cup dried herbs or flowers (your own or shop bought)

250ml (9fl oz) olive, almond or jojoba oil (carrier oil)

210g (7¼oz) cup shea butter (optional)

225g (8oz) cup beeswax

10 drops essential oil, such as frankincense, rosemary or lavender

You will also need

large sterilised glass preserving jar

muslin or cheesecloth

large jar or bowl

non-reactive saucepan or stainless steel double boiler

small sterilised glass jars

pouring jug or funnel

Method

Fill a sterilised jar about three-quarters of the way full with thoroughly dried herbs or flowers, cover in your chosen carrier oil and seal the jar tightly.

Sit the jar on a sunny window sill for 2–3 weeks, shaking every few days. If you see mould growing, it means the herbs/flowers weren't sufficiently dry and you will need to throw it away and start again.

When the infused oil is ready, it should be clear and clean and smell faintly of the herb. Strain out the herbs using some muslin or cheesecloth tied around a jar or bowl, and discard the leftover plant matter.

Now to make the balm, melt the beeswax in a non-reactive stainless steel saucepan or double boiler over a low heat, then add your infused oil and shea butter and stir gently.

When everything is melted together, add your chosen essential oil(s) and stir again to blend them all. Pour into small sterilised glass jars using a pouring jug or funnel and leave for a few hours to cool and harden.

Store in a cool, dry place out of direct sunlight. Enjoy and apply as desired.

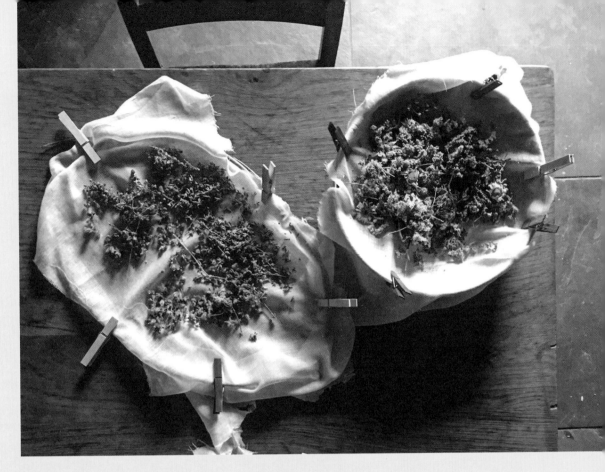

Drying your own flowers and herbs

Collect them on a dry sunny day. If they're damp from dew or rain they are more likely to go mouldy. Ensure, too, that they haven't been sprayed with pesticides, as they will be used on your skin.

Spread out straightaway in a single layer over a clean tea towel or layer of muslin pegged over a basket to allow for good air circulation. Leave in a hot, dry, sunny place. The flowers and herbs are ready when they are completely crumbly dry. In the right conditions this should only take a day or two.

Some herbs and their healing properties

Marigold/calendula is anti-inflammatory and anti-hemorrhagic; helps bind and mend a wound when applied directly; also soothing and moisturising for dry skin.

Yarrow is known to heal rashes and broken skin.

Daisy is anti-inflammatory; used on sores and wounds.

Chamomile is anti-inflammatory; excellent at promoting deep restfulness.

Lavender is calming and relaxing to nervous system; purifying for skin and hair.

Rose is astringent and anti-inflammatory; cools the skin.

fforest tomato ketchup
Storing the summer sunshine in a bottle.

We have a big polytunnel up behind the farmhouse, and every year one whole side is planted with tomatoes and basil. We grow several different types of heritage tomatoes and we love to eat them just as they are with a bit of salt and olive oil. We also send some down to our pizza restaurant, Pizzatipi, in Cardigan for the pizza specials and use them in all manner of ways in cooking. It is a particularly delicious way to savour an intense tomato flavour well into the winter.

This recipe comes from my mother, who can never quite remember how she makes it, so each time it is slightly different. Heather, our cook at fforest, has slightly tweaked it.

Ingredients

1 large red onion, chopped

1 small fennel bulb, trimmed and chopped

1 celery stick, trimmed and chopped

olive oil

1 thumb-sized piece of fresh ginger, peeled and chopped

2 garlic cloves , peeled and chopped

1 red chilli , deseeded and finely chopped

1 bunch basil, leaves picked, stalks chopped

1 tablespoon coriander seeds

2 cloves

2kg (4l 8oz) fresh tomatoes, chopped, (no need to peel or de-seed)

200ml (7fl oz) red wine vinegar

70g (2¼oz) soft brown sugar

sea salt

freshly ground black pepper

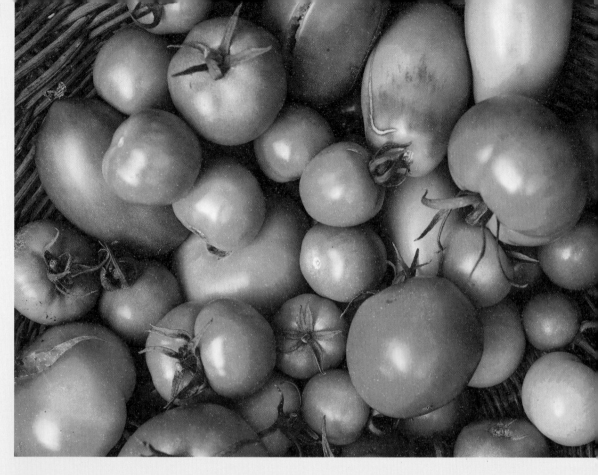

Method

Put the onion, fennel and celery in a large heavy-bottomed saucepan with a big splash of olive oil, the ginger, garlic, chilli, basil stalks, coriander seeds and cloves. Season with salt and pepper.

Cook gently over a low heat for 10–15 minutes, stirring every so often, until the vegetables have softened

Add the tomatoes with 350ml (12fl oz) of cold water. Bring to the boil, then reduce the heat to a simmer and cook gently until the sauce has reduced by half, becoming intensely rich.

Add the basil leaves, then either blitz the sauce in a food processor or in the pan with a hand blender. Push the purée through a sieve set over a bowl twice, to make it really smooth and shiny.

Pour the sauce into a clean pan and add the vinegar and sugar. Bring to a simmer and cook until it has reduced and thickened to the consistency of a luscious tomato ketchup. Taste, and adjust the seasoning if necessary.

Pour the ketchup through a sterilised funnel into sterilised bottles, seal tightly and keep in a cool dark place or in the refrigerator until needed — it should keep for six months.

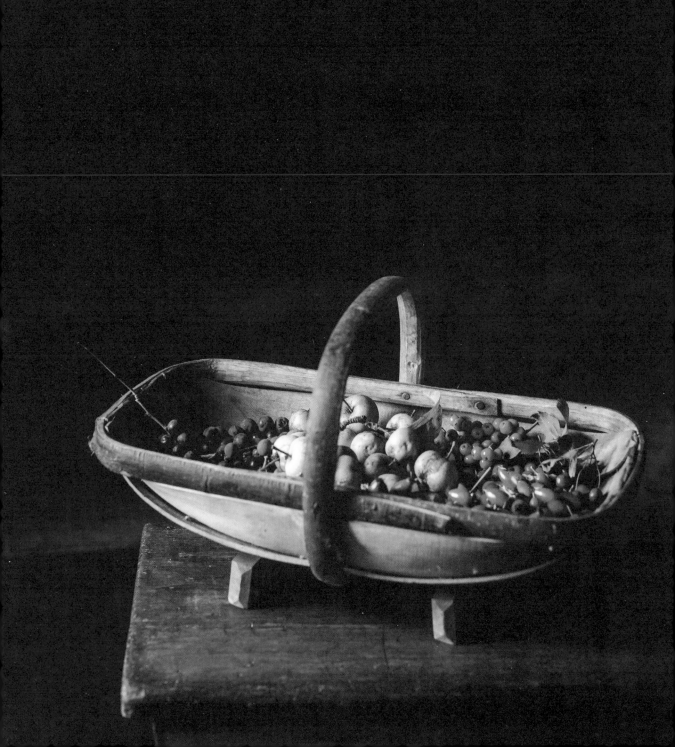

Hedgerow ramble bramble jelly

Double contentment: first the joy of picking and foraging for fruits in the hedgerows; then a delicious jam with a wonderful boost of natural vitamin C to keep away the winter blues.

All these wild autumn hedgerow fruits and berries are low in pectin, which means they need to be combined with the apples to get a good set.

Ingredients

This will give you approximately 8 x 225g (8oz) jars of jelly that will last up to a year in a cupboard (if you haven't eaten it already)

1kg (2lb 4oz) wild crab apples or cooking apples washed and cut into chunks (there's no need to peel or core them as they are going to be strained)

1kg (2lb 4oz) mixture of blackberries, damsons, plums, boysenberries, elderberries, sloes, rosehips (chopped into bits), rowan berries, raspberries, hawthorn berries — a mix of whatever you find on your hedgerow forage, washed

granulated sugar

Method

Put the crab apples, rosehips, sloes, rowan and hawthorn berries and damsons into a preserving pan and cover with water.

Cook slowly over a medium heat for 15 minutes, adding fruits such as blackberries, boysenberries and raspberries during the last 5 minutes of the cooking time as they will soften much more quickly than the others. Cook until everything is pulpy and tender.

Pass the mixture through a jam strainer or a tie up in a muslin suspended over a large bowl for at a least 4 hours or overnight.

Measure the sieved liquid, put it back into the cleaned preserving pan and add 450g (1lb) of sugar for every 600ml (20fl oz) of juice.

Slowly bring to the boil, stirring to dissolve the sugar.

When the sugar has dissolved, boil rapidly for 8–10 minutes, until it reaches setting point.

Test for setting by dropping a spoonful of the mixture onto a cold plate. If it wrinkles when pushed with your finger it is ready.

Leave to cool slightly before pouring into clean and sterilised jars, sealing straight away with lids.

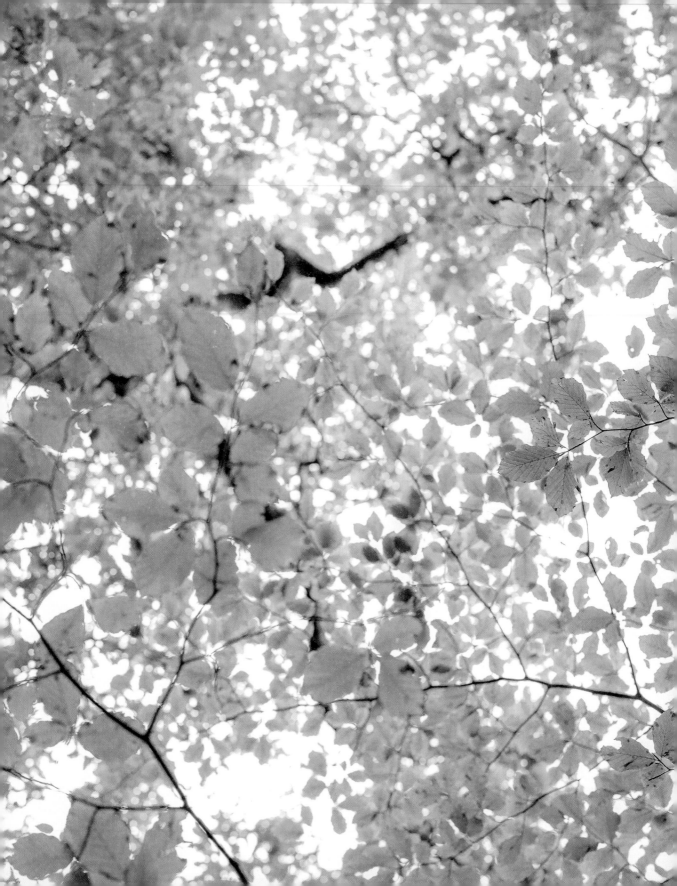

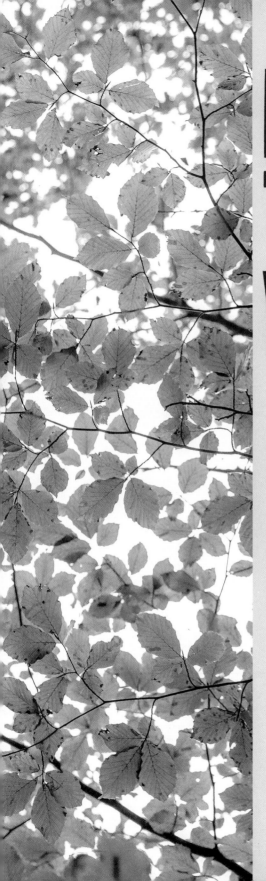

INTO THE WOODS

In nature, nothing is perfect
and everything is perfect.
Alice Walker

Trees appeared on Earth 200,000 years
before humans, and many of these
magnificent plants live for up to six times
longer than the oldest humans.

Trees live by the seasons, wise to changes, and their aim is not
to be happy but to grow. Calmly and passively, with their feet
firmly rooted in the soil, and their arms reaching up to the sky,
trees soak up all the elements, minerals, sunshine and rain. They
produce new growth, strong growth, firm growth. They take time
to rest and let go, shedding leaves and deadwood, adapting to the
weather and environmental conditions.

Even when a tree does finally die, it continues to provide a slow,
steady source of nitrogen, and a home to many creatures, fungi,
mosses and lichens. Power and all respect to trees.

At fforest we are surrounded by ancient oak woods full of twisted,
bent and contorted trees with long branches that have been
allowed to grow naturally for hundreds of years as they feel their
way up to the sunlight. To the south of us, there is a wood of tall
strong pine trees — Douglas fir trunks shooting bolt upright to
the sky, straight as you like, perfect for the ships' masts that, back
in the day when Cardigan was a busy port and harbour, were
used to build boats. Next to the pine wood, towards the village of
Cilgerran, is a coppicing woodland, rich with birch, willow, beech,
sycamore and ash.

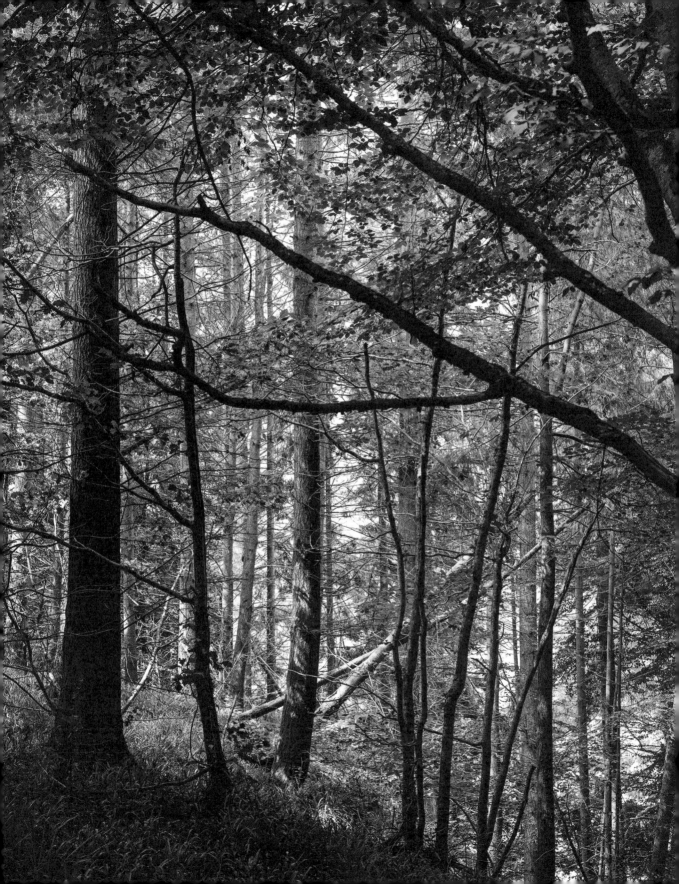

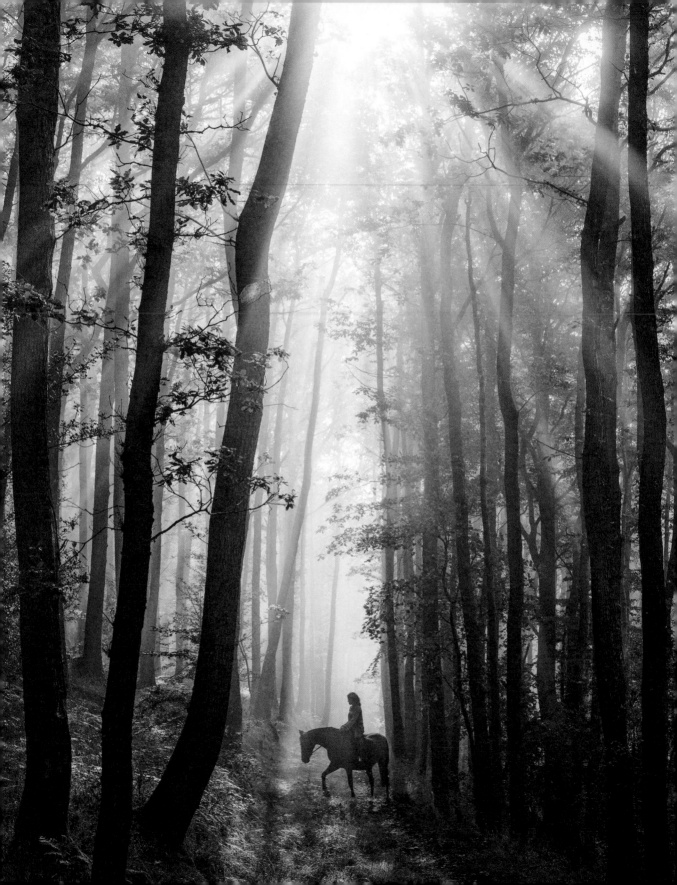

Tree lore

It is not so much for its beauty that the forest makes a claim upon men's hearts, as for that subtle something, that quality of air that emanation from old trees, that so wonderfully changes and renews a weary spirit.
Robert Louis Stevenson

Trees are a truly remarkable and defining feature of our landscape. With their ever-changing beauty, they have covered our landscape for more than a million years. They offer shelter and shade from the elements, are home to many insects and creatures, and are also a source of food and fuel.

In the UK we are lucky to have several ancient woods. The Woodland Trust estimates there are 100,000 ancient trees across Britain, which is believed to be 70 per cent of the European total. The reason these trees have survived is because they were preserved in the estates of the aristocracy and in royal hunting forests. In contrast, our European neighbours harvested their forests for timber.

If trees could talk, there is much these ancient living treasures could tell us about the comings and goings of daily travels through the centuries. Imagine what they might have seen and heard passing and under their leaves and branches, the secrets, dreams, lovers' meetings, gossiping, whispers, crying, planning, plotting and even killings and murders.

Part of the age-old magic of forests lies in the ideas that people have had about trees, the tales, stories and legends. In folklore, forests and woods are mysterious, enchanted places where heroes lose their way, face unexpected challenges and stumble on hidden secrets. They are homes to wolves, witches, wizards, fairies, giants, goblins, dragons, imps, ogres, trolls, unicorns and other supernatural beings. They are wild places of refuge and magic, where imagination and the subconscious can roam free. In these dark places, trees play an important role.

Myths and Legends

I thought all the trees were whispering
to each other, passing news and plots along
in an unintelligible language; and the branches
swayed and groped without any wind.
The Fellowship of the Ring, JRR Tolkein

Many myths and legends from around
the world involve magic trees, talking
trees, trees that act as ladders between
worlds, as sources of life and wisdom.

**In the fairy tales of the
Brothers Grimm**, for
example, Little Red Riding
Hood, with her cloak woven
from wool, dyed bright with
wild red berries, strays from
the path and encounters a
wolf masquerading as her
grandmother.

Hansel and Gretel, the
children of a poor woodcutter,
are left in the woods to
fend for themselves, and
encounter a witch.

Snow White finds a magical
refuge in the woods from her
evil stepmother.

Robin Hood and his band of
merry men find sanctuary in
Sherwood Forest.

Shakespeare's *A
Midsummer Night's Dream*
is set in an enchanted forest.

**In more recent times,
Dorothy** finds herself in a
magical land with animated
trees in The Wizard of Oz.

Tolkien's *Lord of the Rings*
features Forest Fangorn,
home to the tree shepherds.

And in the *Harry Potter*
books there is a forbidden
magical forest near
Hogwarts.

By word of mouth across the
lands, many other wild and
wonderful, dark and often
scary tales of the woods have
been passed down through
the centuries. If ever you
find yourself in the tiny little
stone pub on the edge of our
woods with James, get him to
tell you the fforest ghost story.

Oak

And the wind said, 'May you be as strong as the oak, yet flexible as the birch, may you stand as tall as the redwood, live gracefully as the willow and may you always bear fruit all your days on this earth.'
Native American Prayer

The oak, a large and majestic deciduous tree, is the commonest tree in our shrinking woodlands and is probably the best known and best beloved of all in our British landscape, though it is also widespread in Europe. It grows up to 20–45m (65–150ft) tall and spreads almost as wide.

Oaks can live for up to 1,000 years, though by the time they are 700 years old they have reached old age and afterwards grow only very slowly, sometimes even shrinking to preserve themselves. The saying is that an oak grows for 300 years, is mature for 300 years and takes 300 years to die.

The bark of the oak is very thick and textured, with deep furrows and grooves as if it is wearing a strong jacket of armour. In spring, the trees drip with flowers — long, yellow catkins — and sprout fresh green rounded wavy leaves that have 5–7 lobes on each side and mature to a much darker green as they grow to a length of around 8 cm (3½ in). These leaves fall in autumn as a patchwork of browns, greens and yellows on the ground below, along with the greeny-brown fruits called acorns, wearing the tiny cup-like hats that hold them.

Over its lifetime, an oak will produce as many as 10 million acorns but it has to be at least 40 years old before it starts to do so, with peak production being when the tree is 80–120 years old. Pigs, deer and badgers love to eat acorns, but they are poisonous to horses and cattle. For human consumption they take a fair bit of soaking and preparation to get rid of all the bitterness and poisons. Historically, they were ground up to make an acorn flour for baking bread, cakes and pastries. It has a nutty flavour, although I have never tried it.

The beauty and character of oak has for centuries been preserved in furniture, ships and houses. It cannot be harvested, however, until the tree is 150 years old, making it one of the hardest and most durable timbers on the planet.

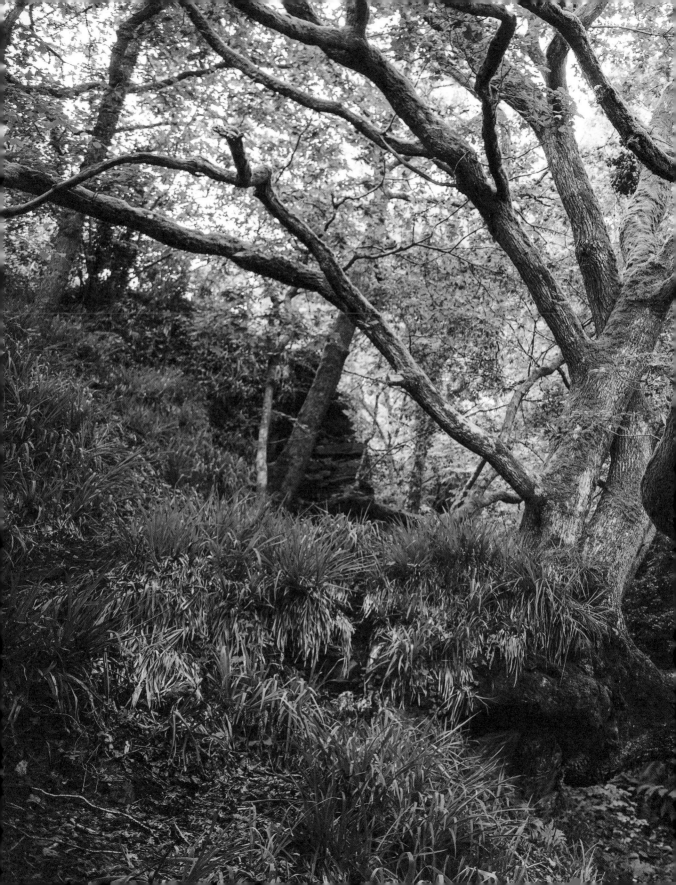

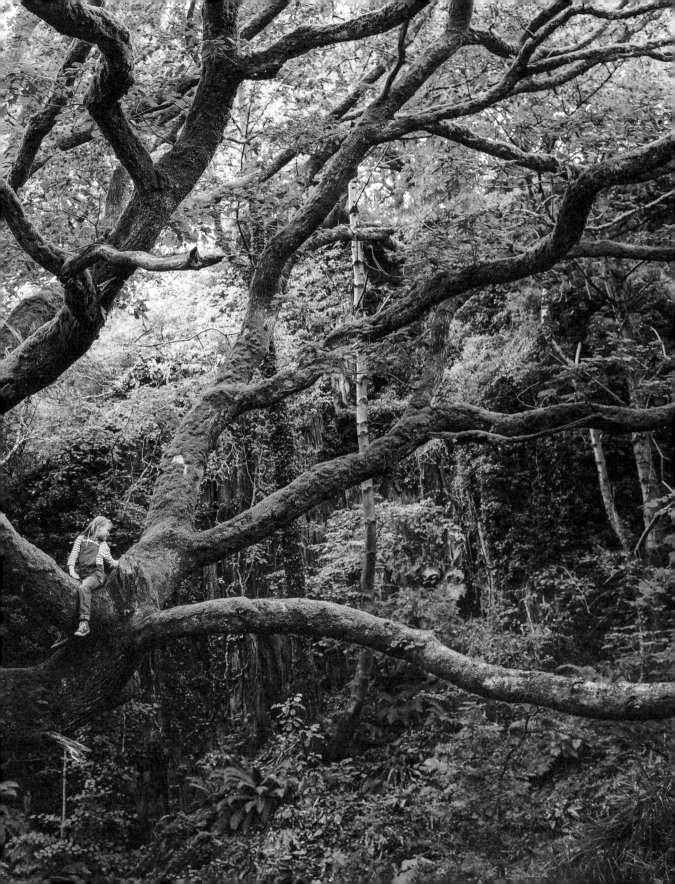

Oak barrels are used for storing wine, whisky and brandy as the wood adds a special aroma and flavour to these drinks. And the tannin found in the bark has been used to treat leather since Roman times.

Heartwood is the dense inner 'heart' of the tree or branch, and is surrounded by the sapwood, via which the sap and nutrients are carried around the tree, which is in turn covered and protected by the bark. At fforest we harvest the standing dead branches of oak, from which time and beetles have removed the sapwood, and use them to make heartwood halos. The branches are harvested only at night on a full moon, and when assembled they are hung in the farmhouse where they emit the soft glow of the captured moonlight (assisted by some discreet LEDs).

Oak apples, also known as galls, are round, crab apple-like growths, 2–4cm (¾–1½in) in diameter, that have been used to make writing ink since the Middle Ages, and well into the early twentieth century.

Throughout Europe, the oak is known as the tree of the thunder gods, as it is the tree most commonly struck by lightning.

Merlin's Oak is said to have grown from an acorn planted by the magician on the outskirts of a town near fforest called Carmarthen. Merlin put a protective spell on it, predicting disaster to the town if it was ever felled. By the time I was a child, all that remained of the tree was a blackened trunk preserved behind iron railings. It was finally moved at the end of the 1970s and put into the town's museum, whereupon Carmarthen suffered its worst floods for many years.

Beech

The clearest way into the Universe
is through a forest wilderness.
John Muir

The beautiful, tall and stately beech is attractive throughout the year. In early spring the pointed red buds open to reveal young tender lime green leaves with silky hairs, which darken and toughen up as they mature. The simple, ovalish-shaped leaves, which grow to between 4–9cm (1½–3¾in) long, have wavy edges that appear almost corrugated and lead to point at the tip. When autumn arrives, the leaves turn a most beautiful golden, coppery, rust colour — an uplifting sight when the shimmering sun shines through them. As the year progresses, the dead, crackly, bleached-brown leaves can stay clinging onto their twigs, rattling in the wind throughout the winter before they finally fall.

Small yellowish-green flowers appear as the leaves unfurl from the buds in the spring. These flowers then transform into prickly green husks that contain shiny brown nuts. As the husks dry, bristle, brown and go woody, it splits releasing the beech nuts in the autumn. Beechmast is the collective term for beech nuts.

Beech can live for a long time, sometimes more than 1,000 years. As a result, they make a brilliant habitat for many hole-nesting birds and wood-boring insects. The smooth grey bark is also a popular place for a complex flora of different fungi, mosses and lichens that pepper a camouflage patina of texture and colour up the trunk and branches.

As beech trees are shallow rooted and tall, mature trees, which can grow up to 40m (130ft), are at risk of being uprooted in high winds. Sadly, in the Great Storm of 1987, which badly hit southern England, beech trees took the brunt and thousands of mature trees fell.

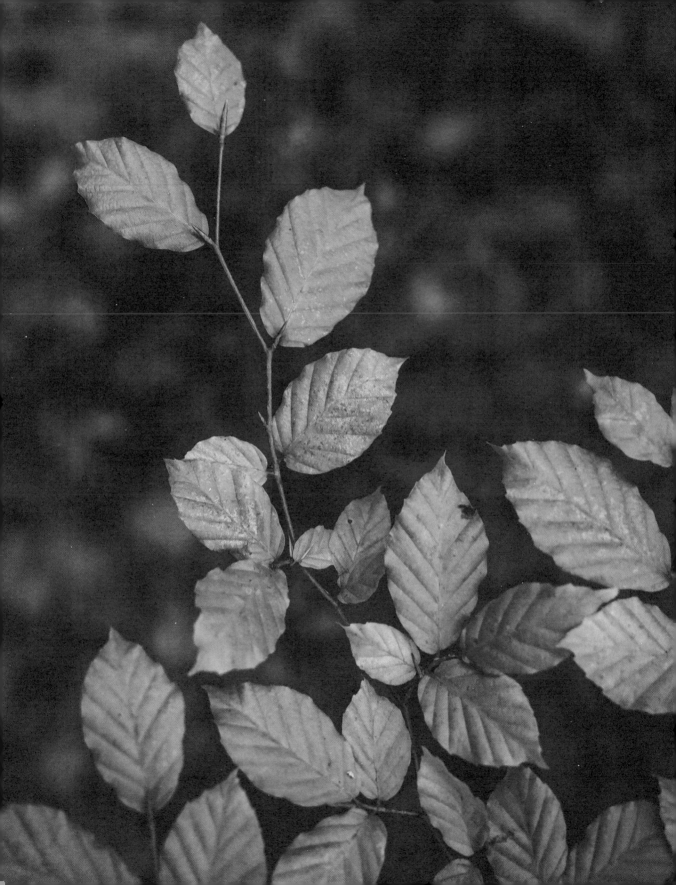

Beech leaf noyau

Noyau is a brandy liqueur flavoured with almonds and apricot stones that has been made at Poissey in northern central France since the early nineteenth century. For this version, it's best to use inexpensive neutral-flavoured gin, as the flavour of more expensive kinds can compete with the citrus of the beech leaves.

The brandy can be omitted but it adds a rich note. Use more or less sugar according to your preference. Mine is for less sweet, though the amount of sugar in the recipe is for middle sweet liqueur.

Ingredients

approx. 400g young beech leaves (enough so the gin just covers them)

700ml (1¼ pints) gin

150g (5½ oz) white sugar

40ml (1½ fl oz) brandy

Method

Gather young, soft, bright green beech leaves. Remove any twigs. Lightly pack enough leaves in a jar so that the gin just covers them. Seal the jar and leave standing in a dark cool place for a minimum of a month (two months is even better). After this time, strain through a fine muslin, squeeze out the leaves and discard to the compost.

In a saucepan, dissolve the sugar in 300ml (½ pint) of water over a gentle heat. It is important to make sure the sugar is completely dissolved. Once cool, add this syrup to the infused gin, then add the brandy and decant into a bottle. The liqueur can be drunk any time from then but will continue to mature and become more rounded the longer you leave it. Ideally, wait for a minimum of three months, if you can resist.

Sycamore

A tree of good luck, bad luck and creativity,
it is now a part of us.
Egyptian creation myth

These massive, fast-growing broad-leaved trees are loved for their shade. Sycamores can grow to 35m (115 feet) and can live for 400 years. They are relatively new to the British landscape; they were introduced from Europe during the Middle Ages and spread rapidly across the landscape.

Sycamores are wonderfully hardy and robust trees and grow in places that would stunt most others. They thrive in wet and wind-swept, salt-laden air, so are happy on the coast and have a mass of wonderfully delicate and intricate flowers that dangle like little lanterns in spring.

They are probably best known for their helicopter-winged seeds that playfully spin and fly to earth in the autumn.

The sycamore bark is smooth and grey when young, but as the tree grows and matures the bark becomes rough and brittle with age, creating a distinctive pattern of browns, greens and greys. The bark can't cope with the rapid growth that the sycamores experience, which means the bark frequently peels off, resulting in a patchy, flaky appearance when the younger bark beneath is revealed.

The twigs grow off the branches in one direction, then switch directions just after a bud growth, creating a zig-zag shape. A sycamore has large dark green, raggedy edged leaves that have three to five pointed lobes. Leathery in texture, they have thick veins protruding on the underside. I especially love the stalks as they are often tinged a pinky red.

The wood is hard and strong, creamy-white with a fine grain. The wood does not taint or stain with food, which makes it perfect for making furniture, kitchenware. It is also used to make musical instruments.

The wood is excellent for carving, and in Wales it is the wood that is traditionally used for making love spoons, a hand-carved gift given to a young woman by her suitor.

Ash

In Norse mythology, the ash is seen as the world tree Yggdrasil, or Cosmic Ash.

Ash trees are tall and graceful and can live for 400 years, often growing to a height of 35m (115ft). They love deep, well -drained soil and a cool atmosphere, and as a result often dominate British woodlands. (We have a lot of them here at fforest.) They are a common and widespread tree of northern Europe and Asia and parts of Africa.

The bark is pale brown to grey in colour, often with a beautiful patina of lichen and mosses.

The feathery leaves can be confused with those of the smaller rowan tree, whose leaves are serrated, or an elder, which has fewer leaflets. The common ash leaves are a rich green colour and they are amongst the last leaves to appear on the trees in the spring and the last to drop in the autumn.

Ash is an easy tree to recognise, even in winter, long after the leaves have fallen, as bunches of the brown-winged seeds, commonly called ash keys, cling and hang below the branches and don't fall until the spring.

Ash wood is both very strong and elastic. It is one of the toughest hardwoods; it absorbs shocks without splintering and it is said that a joint of ash will bear more weight than any other wood, which makes it the perfect wood for the handles of all kinds of tools, including hammers, axes and spades. In times gone by, it was a mainstay for making bows and spears, wheel axles, wagons and carriages and more recently has been used to make tennis rackets, hockey sticks and oars.

Silver birch

In early Celtic mythology, the birch symbolised renewal and purification, love and fertility.

An elegant and graceful tree with thin branches and twigs that droop and bend downwards, the silver birch has distinctive white peeling papery bark. In summer they are covered with delicate, light green, triangular-shaped serrated leaves, creating a light open canopy above, which allow the perfect conditions on the ground for grass, moss and all spring flowers to grow underneath.

The birch is relatively fast growing, reaching up to 30m (100ft) in height. It grows in a wide range of temperatures, from Lapland to the Mediterranean, although it thrives best in the woodlands and forests of Russia, America and Scandinavia, where it grows higher up mountains than any other deciduous tree.

Birch bark stays white all year-round. Light and strong, it was used by Native Americans to make canoes, which they made more waterproof with pitch from pine trees. Birch bark has also been used for shelters and to write on and to make tar oil.

Bundles of twigs can be made into a broom, which was traditionally used to sweep out the spirits of the old year, and to cleanse negative energies out of a room. Some gardeners still like to use a birch broom, known as a besom broom, to 'purify' their gardens.

Every autumn birch trees collect and store summer nutrients in their roots to help with new tree growth in the spring. After the long cold freezing winter, as the days starts to warm up and the freezing ground begins to thaw, the sap rises and flows from the roots up the tree. For just two or three weeks of the year in early spring, hundreds of litres of sap rises daily, pouring up the mature birch trees. This birch water, which we first tasted at the restaurant Noma in Copenhagen, is considered to be a tonic after a long cold dark winter. Smooth and silky, it tastes similar to a light watery clear maple syrup and has been drunk for hundreds for years in Russia, Scandinavia and in the Baltics as an anti-inflammatory and cleansing supplement.

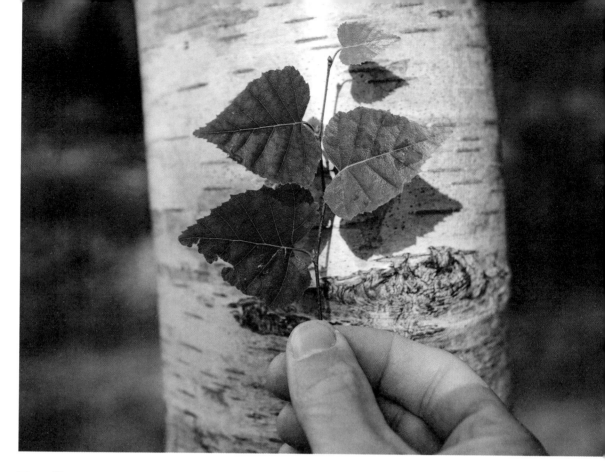

To collect it the sap, a spout is inserted into a hole drilled into the tree and the spout directs the sap into a bucket. This sap can be drunk fresh as a spring tonic, used in place of water to make tea and coffee, made into carbonated drinks, beer and wine or boiled down to make syrup. The sap water should be kept cool in a refrigerator for no more than six days, or it can be frozen for future use. The window for collecting the sap is only a few weeks each spring, as root pressure changes and when leaves begin to develop the sap stops flowing. Choose mature birch trees that are 20cm (8in) in diameter or larger to tap. Place only one tap in a tree each year.

To cool any violent passion, anger or overreaction, sit alone for a while with your back against a birch trunk. If this isn't possible, take something of birch in your hands and sit alone and quiet. Its innocent energy will channel your strong feelings into wise ways.

Holly

Holly was seen as a fertility symbol and a charm against witches, goblins and the devil.

A much-loved, conical-shaped, gorgeous, glossy evergreen tree, holly is easily identified by its bright-red berries and dark green, shiny and spiky leaves, which have long been used to decorate homes in winter. Pulling on wellies and wrapping up warm to walk out into the woods and collect holly and ivy is such an immensely happy and festive thing to do. However, holly trees don't produce their jewel-like, bright-red berries until they have been growing for around 40 years, and the berries only adorn the female trees. For many hungry birds in winter holly berries are a mainstay of their diet, but please don't eat them yourself, as they are poisonous to humans. Even a small amount can make you very ill, and if you ingest more than 20 berries it could be fatal.

A mature tree can grow up to 15m (50ft) and live for 300 years. The bark is smooth and thin. It is the younger plants that have the spiky leaves, those in the upper parts of older trees are more likely to be smooth and oval. The thick and waxy surface of the leaves helps the tree to resist water loss. The leaves can last up to four years on the tree, which explains how sprigs and wreathes can also survive the festive season. Tiny four-petalled white flowers arrive in the spring.

The Oak and Holly Kings are twin brothers and also old enemies, but despite their enmity they are not complete without each other. At the beginning of the year, at the Winter Solstice (21 December), or Yule in the Wheel of the Year, the Oak King battles with Holly and defeats him. Oak now can rule the first half of the year, as the Sun waxes and grows in strength and the light lengthens. **At the Summer Solstice** (21 June), or Litha in the Wheel of the Year, the brothers battle again. This time Holly triumphs. In the old tradition, the body of Oak was burnt on the Summer Solstice fire. Now, as the days get darker and shorter and the Sun loses its strength, Holly rules until the year turns once again towards the light. **The brothers don't die in the battles** for the light and dark but go back to the astral plane to serve the Goddess Arianrhod at her silver star wheel, and await the times for their solstice re-incarnation.

Rowan

Throughout Europe the rowan was considered sacred and was widely venerated as the tree of strongest possible protection over malicious, magical influences.

This small, graceful, bright and open tree with smooth, grey-brown bark is loved for its pretty creamy-white frothing clusters of flowers in May, followed by large bunches of brilliantly bright red and orange berries from late August. These berries are loved by all the birds — especially blackbirds — so don't last long on the tree. They are edible for humans too. They are very sour but rich in vitamin C and can be turned into a delicious jelly, perfect to accompany meats. If you do want to make a jelly with them you'd better pick them pretty quickly.

The serrated feather-like leaves made up of eight pairs of long, oval and toothed leaflets turn from deep green in summer to bright red and golden orange in the autumn before they finally fall.

The rowan is a fairly short-lived deciduous tree, not reaching much above 15m (50ft). It is extremely hardy, in fact one of the hardiest European trees. A rowan is happy in poor soil, living on a rocky mountain side and surviving icy temperatures, making it a true Celtic native of Wales and Scotland, which explains why it's sometimes known as the mountain ash.

The rowan loves light and space so it doesn't grow well in old woodlands or forests where it is overshadowed by much taller oaks and pines.

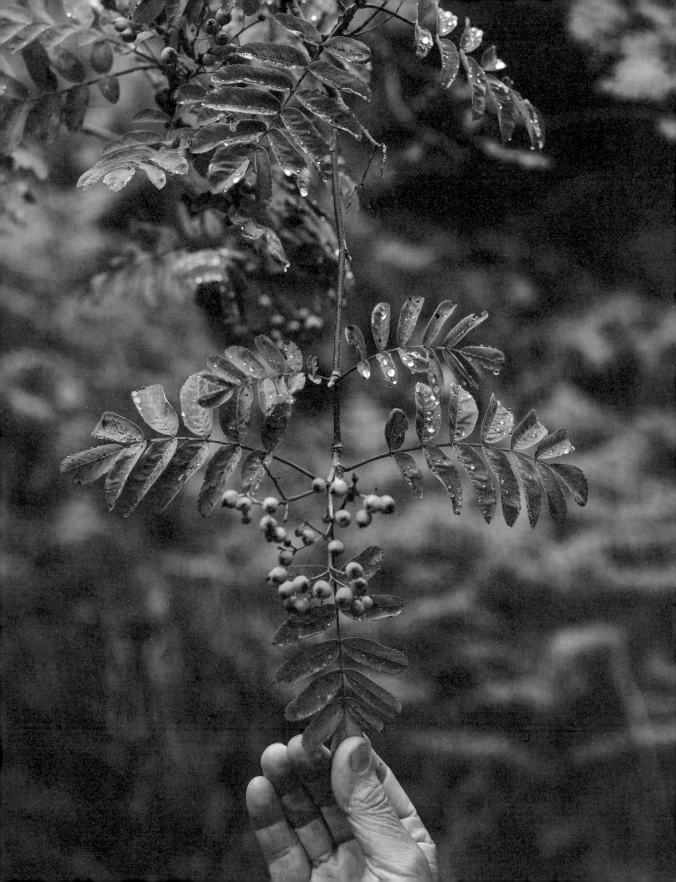

Elder

It is considered unlucky to cut down an elder.
If you must do it, ask permission respectfully
of the tree and explain why it's necessary!
Give the spirit time to move before cutting and
never bring the wood into the house to burn.

A smallish tree that loves light and grows best in slightly damp, fertile soil, elder is often found by roadsides and along banks where rabbits, badgers and foxes root and dig around. In late spring it has huge creamy white saucers of tiny-petalled flowers, anything up to 20cm (8in) across, that are used to make cordial. The flowers are followed in autumn by masses of small, purplish-black berries, hanging off long stalks, which are used to make wine and jam and flavour gin. But beware: the unripe green berries are poisonous. Traditionally, having a rowan by the front of your house and an elder near the back gave protection to your home.

The bark is quite rough and brittle, but the stems are soft and filled with a white pith that's easily removed and hollowed out. For centuries elder wood has been used to make whistles, musical pipes and beads.

Elder wood itself makes a very poor fuel; the structure of the wood and its sap makes it scream and spit whilst burning, giving the belief that it was the Devil spitting from the heat of the fire.

The name elder means 'fire' It comes from the Anglo-Saxon 'aeld' and was so called because the hollow stems were used as bellows to blow air into the centre of a fire.

A string of elder beads offers protection from angry spirits, either when worn or hung outside a back door.

Elderflower cordial

Freshly picked flowers make the best cordial. Gather on a warm dry day — the flowers should be white and fresh and smell of lemon. Make sure you have time to make the cordial after picking, as the flowers lose their fresh perfume within a few hours.

Ingredients

Makes about 2 litres (3½ pints)

about 25–30 heads of elderflower blossom

finely grated zest of 3 unwaxed lemons and their juice

2kg (4lb 4oz) of white sugar

1 heaped teaspoon citric acid (optional)

Method

Gently heat the sugar and 1.5 litres (2¾ pints) of water together in a saucepan until the sugar has dissolved, stirring occasionally, bring to the boil and then remove from the heat.

Carefully inspect the elderflower heads and shake to remove any insects.

Add the flower heads to the sugar syrup together with the lemon zest, lemon juice and citric acid, if using.

Cover and leave to cool, steep and infuse overnight or for up to 36 hours.

Drain the syrup through a piece of muslin or a very fine sieve.

Using a sterilised funnel, carefully pour the syrup into sterilised bottles.

Seal the bottles with sterilised lids and keep in the refrigerator for up to 6 weeks. Alternatively, you can freeze the cordial in ice cubes.

Delicious served with sparkling water or sparkling wine and goes perfectly with strawberries and rhubarb.

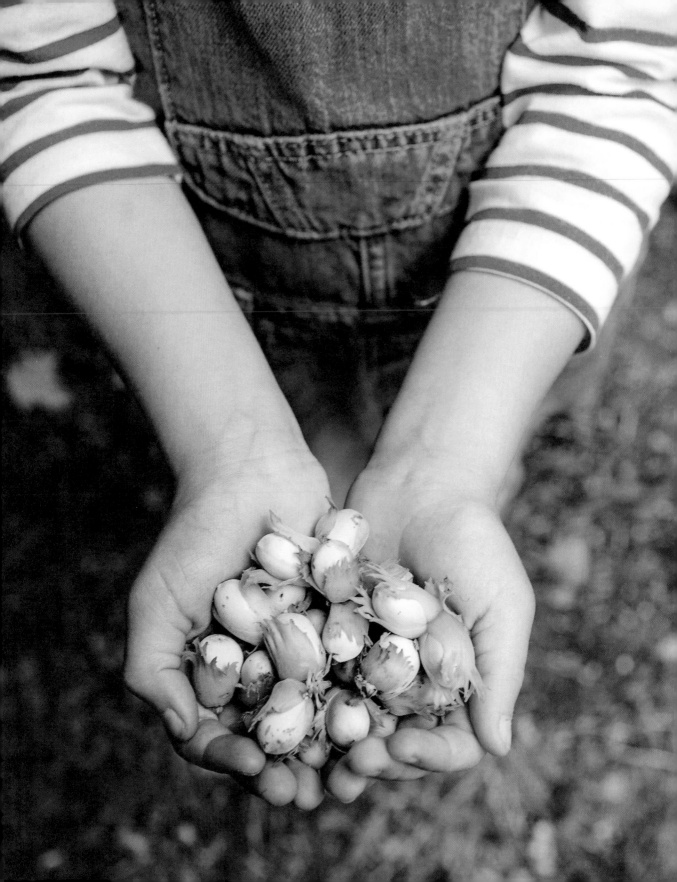

Hazel

The Celts equated hazelnuts with concentrated wisdom and poetic inspiration. A wand or staff made from hazel withy was often chosen by Druid priests. Hazel is associated with the ability to find hidden sources of water and lost items, and was linked to protection and fertility.

The hazel catkin is one of the first things to flower in spring, right at the end of winter. The long pale yellow, frilly and papery male catkin are what you see dangling from the bare twigs. The little wood behind our pub where the fire pit sits is full of hazel trees growing as clumps of slender trunks, but managing to still look like one trunk and canopy tree shape. A hazel leaf is simple, rounded and feels soft and slightly furry. The catkin is the flower and the fruit is the hazelnut. Unfortunately, we don't often get to gather and eat the delicious hazelnuts at fforest before the squirrels do. As they are high in protein and are a really good source of well-flavoured vitamin E, it is no wonder the squirrels love them.

Hazel responds to coppicing, a practice which can actually extend and even double the lifespan of the tree. The long, thin and straight shoots that grow up from the base of the tree are called withies. They are very pliable and are cut for walking sticks and natural fencing, and can even be pinned into shape while still growing. Long ago, they were widely used to form the wattle in wattle-and-daub buildings.

Hawthorn

The Welsh Goddess Olwen, the White Goddess of the Hawthorn, once walked the empty universe and her white track of hawthorn petals became the Milky Way.

The star-shaped flowers of the hawthorn, which are white, speckled with pink, blossom after the tree's leaves have unfurled. The hawthorn is at its most prominent in the British landscape when it blossoms during the month of May, which gives rise to its common name: the May tree. It has many associations with May Day festivities where the blossoms were used for garlands and for decorations outside — to this day there is a very strong taboo against bringing hawthorn into the house, except it seems OK to bring it in to eat the edible parts!

Hawthorn leaves are smallish and lobed with jagged edges. The tender young leaves, flower buds and young flowers in spring are edible and are both pretty and delicious when added to a spring green salad. The thorns are short, and the branches are often dense and tangled. The fruits in autumn are bright-red, small beads known as haws. These are not eaten raw as they don't taste very nice and may also cause mild stomach upset, but they can be cooked and are most commonly used to make jellies, wines and ketchups.

Blackthorn

At the Winter Solstice, blackthorn wood is given as an offering to the Underworld powers for the return of the Sun.

The blackthorn, or sloe bush, can often get muddled up with hawthorn as they are similarly thorny, have a very similar flower and are of a similar size. One way to tell the difference is that the blackthorn flowers before the hawthorn, very early in spring, and has a cloud of creamy white starry blossom with tiny orange blobs when the leaves are nothing but tiny buds. It looks just like snow against the black bark of its bare branches.

Blackthorn leaves are quite different to the hawthorn. They are oval and tough, with a very tiny serrated edge. The fruits in autumn are sloe berries, little dark purple ovals, that pepper the branches from late summer. These berries are very bitter until they have been caught by the first heavy frost of winter. They taste awful raw, straight off the tree, and are not ever good to eat — they will make your face pucker up if you try — but when steeped in gin with added sugar for a good few months they make a really delicious fireside tipple for the long, dark, winter evenings.

Blackthorn is known for its long thorns, which are very strong and very sharp. These regularly stick out from their dense and tangled branches and it is very painful if you get scraped. The thorns combined with its tangled branches make blackthorn a perfect natural barrier for keeping livestock in a field. It is pretty hardy and can withstand very strong winds and will thrive in almost any soil.

Blackthorn is an ideal safe space for birds to live and nest in the protective thickets, making it an important haven for wildlife. The leaves provide food for the caterpillars of hairstreak butterflies, which are rare and protected. After an inspector visited us, we were happy to discover we have a thriving colony of hairstreaks in our blackthorn swathes at fforest.

Tree climbing
All our wisdom is stored in the trees.
Santosh Kalwar

Climbing a tree, being held by the strong branches in the canopy, feeling empowered by being up so high where the birds hang out, nest and feel safe and the squirrels look down at the world below, is one of the simplest forms of pleasure.

When we were children and out on adventures we didn't think twice about scrambling up a tree to pick plums or apples or lash up some rope to make a swing. When I was young I was told to be outside all the time, to go out to play and have adventures. I was given the freedom to explore and so I spent a lot of time outside playing and climbing trees. Now, in the main, our children are kept on a much tighter leash by their parents and have sadly become much more used to a safe and sedentary lifestyle indoors, spending more time looking at screens. Many children have become fearful of challenging themselves physically.

Here at fforest we have some majestic beech trees at the back of the farmhouse, and its up these trees that we get Bobby and his brothers, (professional tree surgeons), to set up the ropes and harnesses for tree climbing a few times a year.

Ascending one of these trees provides the excitement of the climb, a wonderful feeling of joy at reaching the top and a calmness at being high in the canopy of a tall tree. There is also such an immense sense of achievement and satisfaction for having done it.

Not only is climbing trees brilliant fun for all, it is great for fitness, coordination, spatial awareness, flexibility, balance and concentration — you are continually problem solving and planning your route. And pretending you are Tarzan!

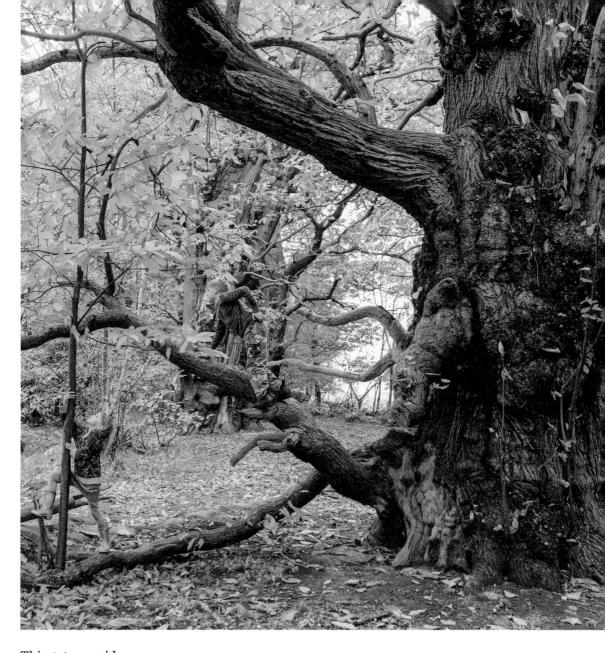

Things to consider

Tree climbing is a risky for any inexperienced tree climber. If you have no prior climbing experience, it is advisable to take a climbing course before going out on your own.

Take the time to learn about the equipment you need to make sure you are safe, and familiarise yourself with advice and guidance on which trees are the best to climb, what is a healthy tree, how to look for potential hazards and how to judge if a branch is large enough to take your weight.

Building a den

A wild animal's hidden home, a lair, a sett, lodge, cave, nest, burrow, dugout, a shelter to be dry, a hidey-hole to be warm and safe, a place to retreat to and relax, somewhere to be cosy and quiet, a place for children to play in their own little space and get lost in their imaginations.

Playing in and making a den is the essence of childhood. It is such brilliant fun and so important for their creativity and development. It could be a hideaway in the garden, a tree house, a living willow dome or a stick and leaf shelter in the woods. A towel, deckchair and windbreak haven on a beach, a cardboard box construction in the living room, retreat under the kitchen table surrounded by chairs and covered with blankets and an old curtain, or a tipi made from long sticks and draped with old sheets. There are so many possibilities for making a den.

At fforest in the summer we build wild dens out in the woods using only the natural materials to be found. Everyone loves to join in, it is a great thing for families to do together to bond and learn real survival skills, problem solving, team work. Creating and learning about different materials and the natural environment. About making a structure.

A den is a frame and a cover. The smaller it is, the warmer and more stable it will be, so please don't get carried away making a house. Here are some tips on building a den.

Method

Find either a fallen tree or a tree with a low branch that can act as a good roof support.

Surround this with branches and sticks to build up the frame and structure — willow and hazel are strong and flexible, but most small branches and twigs will do.

For a natural structure, you can collect leaves, ferns and moss for your roof and walls, remembering to be careful as these are the habitats and homes for many little woodland creatures.

For something more permanent, use a cover, such as a tarpaulin, for the roof and to cover the main frame — this is what many of the world's nomads and explorers would do and it is the one essential item that they carry with them on their travels.

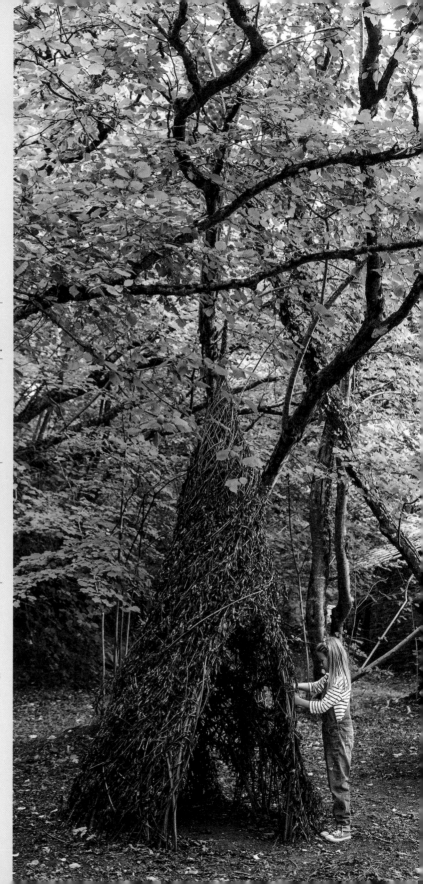

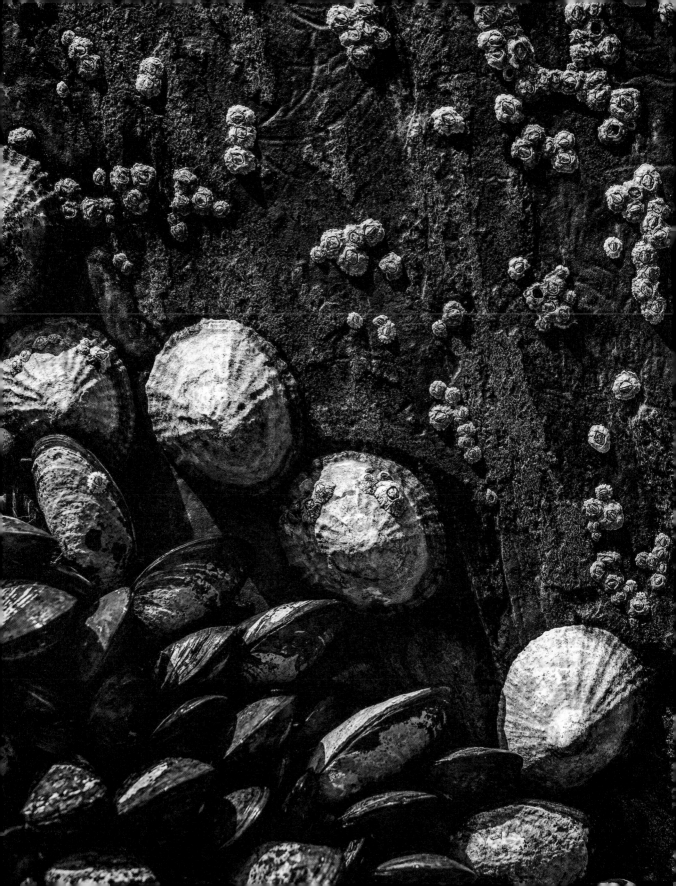

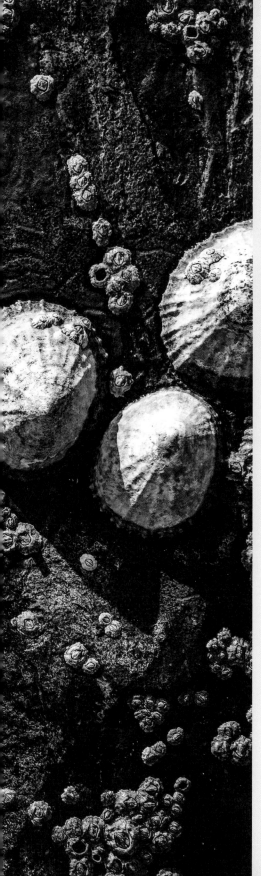

BY THE WATER

On the river

Serene and beautiful, rivers offer
a quieter but no less entrancing
experience as the sea. Paddle, glide
and meander where the water glints,
sparkles, glimmers and shimmers.
Drift under the trees, float into
tranquil pools and eddies. See and
be in those parts of the river that
are invisible from the riverbank.
Paddle upstream in a canoe (which
does require some coordination and
teamwork) then turn and float with
the leaves, rush over rapids, bob with
the ripples, drift with the flow. Look
out for a long-legged heron, a flash of
iridescent kingfisher, flitting dragonfly,
dabbling ducks or a playful otter.

Paddling on the river is a brilliant
way to experience nature with friends
and family. It is also a great way to
stay fit and healthy. However, it can
also be a dangerous activity. River
levels can rise and fall quickly in wet
or dry conditions and present unseen
dangers, so be sure you stay safe.

Water safety

**Before you go out on any
water**, always check the tide
tables and water current,
the safety of the flow and
the water height. Have the
correct safety equipment, a
rope and life jackets. Always
let someone know when and
where you are going, always
call them when you return
back to shore.

There is no rushing a river. When you go there, you go at the pace of the water and that pace ties you into a flow that is older than life on this planet. Acceptance of that pace, even for a day, changes us, reminds us of other rhythms beyond the sound of our own heartbeats.
River Days, Jeff Rennicke

Canoes, kayaks and paddleboards

Canoes are light-framed open boats, tapering to a point at both ends. They are powered by paddlers who kneel on the bottom of the boat, or sit on a raised seat, and propel themselves forward with a single-bladed paddle. A canoe is open topped and it is often referred to as a Canadian canoe. They were traditionally made from dug or burnt-out tree trunks and covered with birch bark, skins or canvas. These days they are usually made of aluminium, fibreglass or moulded plastic.

Kayaks are small and long. They originate from Greenland, and are similar to canoes, though slightly narrower, and with an enclosing deck, to keep out waves and water spray. The paddler sits facing forward with their legs forward, too, and uses a two-bladed paddle on alternate sides to propel themselves through the water.

A sit-on-top kayak has a similar hull shape to a traditional kayak but instead of sitting inside, you sit in a moulded seat on top.

Paddleboards, also known as stand up paddleboards (SUP) are an offshoot of surfing, where a boarder stands on the board — a much bigger, wider, sturdier board than a surfboard — and uses a long single-bladed paddle to propel themselves through the water.

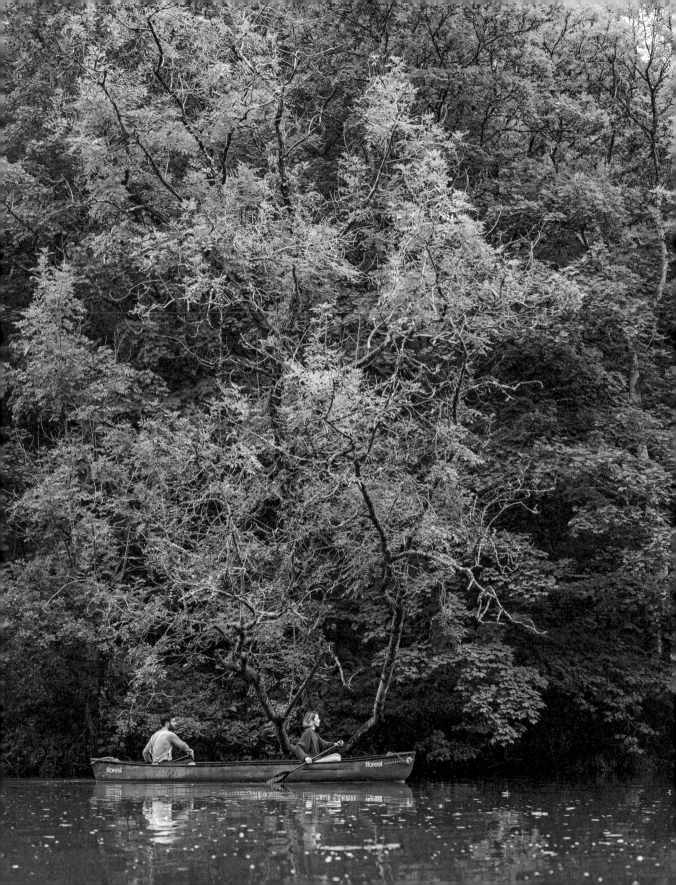

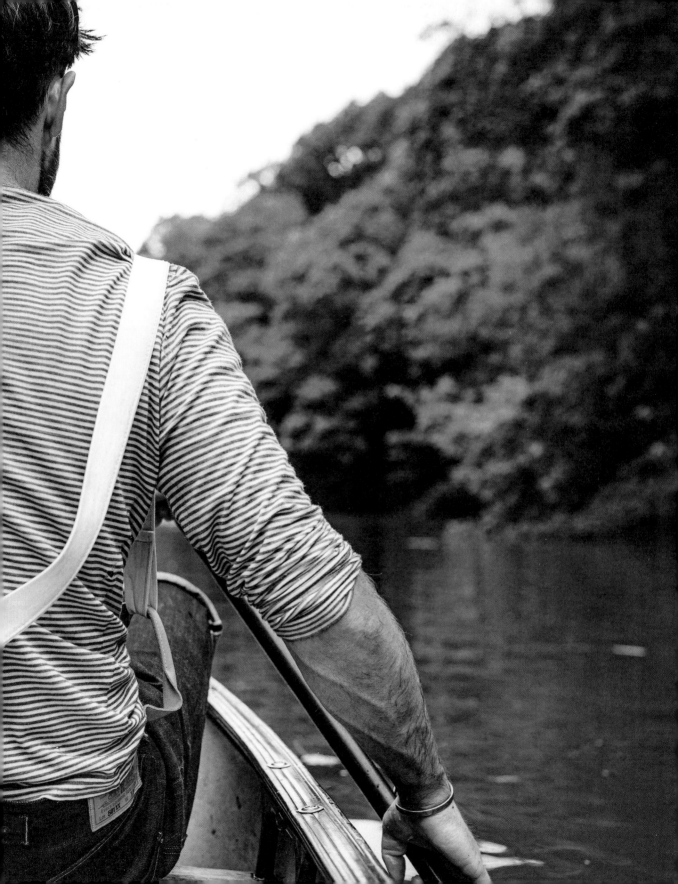

Wild swimming

For whatever we lose (like a you or a me)
It's always ourselves we find in the sea.
E.E. Cummings

At fforest, we're both near to the sea and right next to the beautiful Teifi, the river after which we named our fourth son. Swimming out in these wild and natural waters, surrounded by nature — the trees, the birds, the fresh air — is so liberating and exhilarating, it is something we encourage as it makes you feel so alive.

Any swimming, though, be it plodding up and down in a swimming pool or the freedom of the wilder sea, is very good for you and a great way to exercise. By its repetitive nature it is incredibly meditative. Just as when you are walking or jogging, your breathing becomes regular and deep.

It was here in Wales, in these salty waters, in Aberporth Bay to be precise, that I took my first strokes and felt the magical, floaty feeling of my toes not touching the sand anymore and the amazingly liberating feeling of bobbing in an enormous expanse of moving, living water. When I think back to my childhood, it feels as though much of the summers were spent frolicking in the waves, body-surfing or scrambling over the rocks and diving off high ledges into the sparkling sea. Whatever the weather, we went in the sea, teeth chattering for ages, staying in until our fingers puckered. And the experience still remains to this day totally invigorating.

If you feel lacklustre, grumpy, overwhelmed or uninspired before you go for a swim, everything will feel so much better and clearer afterwards. You never regret going in. However, it is so much easier said than done to muster the courage to plunge into the cold water. Every tiny bit of you is telling you not to do this mad act, which is sometimes quite a painful sensation, but a release of natural endorphins is triggered once you have done it and will make you feel vital and amazing. Swimming in cold water increases the blood flow to your skin, thereby flushing impurities out and improving skin tone. It also soothes achy muscles and boosts the immune system.

When your face and head go into cool water it triggers a mammalian reflex, which is what gives us the tingling feeling at the back of the neck. It also slows our heart rate by 10 per cent, redistributing higher levels of blood to the vital organs. In short, it prepares us for longer submersion, and will keep us alive for longer if we are drowning. Humans and other mammals all have this mammalian response or diving reflex, which is triggered specifically when our face is submerged in water and not just our bodies. The diving reflex is particularly strong in aquatic mammals, such as seals, otters and dolphins, but also exists to a lesser extents in other animals, including humans, particularly babies up to six months old. The moral of this story is that when swimming in the wild, always stick your head in the water to start.

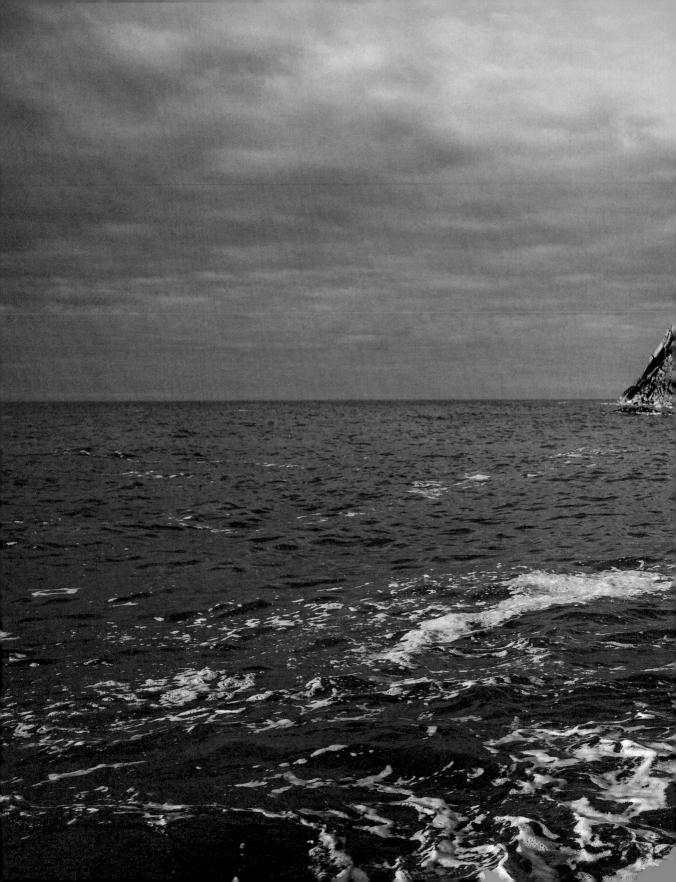

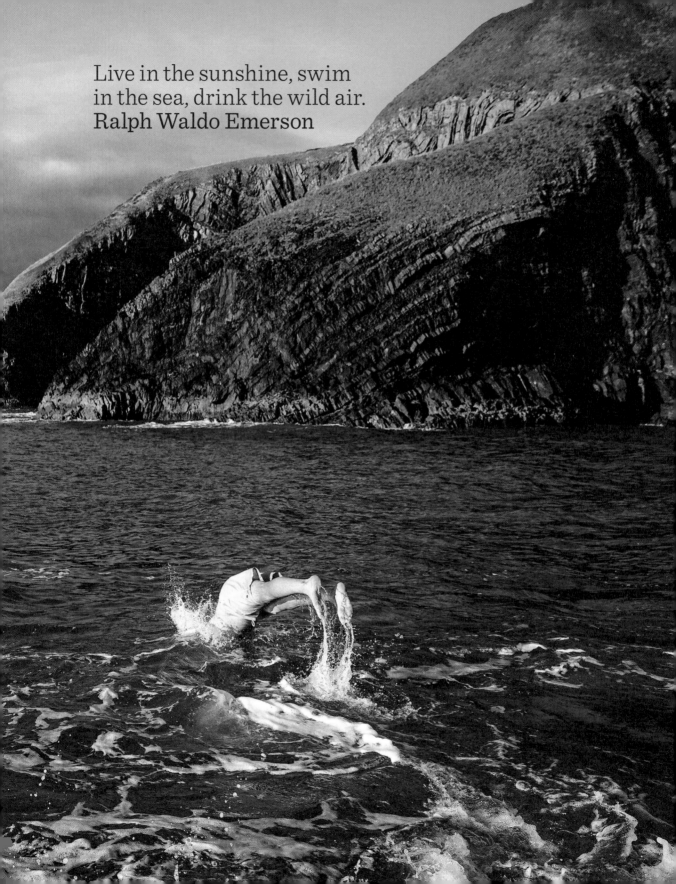

Live in the sunshine, swim
in the sea, drink the wild air.
Ralph Waldo Emerson

At the beach

The cure for anything is salt water:
sweat, tears or the sea.
Isak Dinesen

The oceans cover 71 per cent of the Earth's surface. These immense expanses of salty water can be raging one moment, tranquil and shimmering the next. The daily tidal movements and rhythms are both completely relaxing and totally stimulating. A trip to the sea is blissful, a chance to stop, gaze and daydream, to let yourself go and completely unwind, to hear the waves crashing against the rocks or calmly caressing the sand.

A beach is a place of happy carefree memories, somewhere to run barefoot, skim stones, let the sand tickle between your toes, paddle in the shallows, hear the laughing seagulls, build sandcastles, read a book, fish, snorkel and swim. Laying on the beach, letting the fresh sea air fill your lungs, while soaking up the sunshine, all while getting a good healthy dose of vitamin D, is a brilliant boost for mood, mind and body.

On this far western edge of Wales there is a stunning coastal footpath that weaves its way from the very north of Wales, where it meets the English border, to the very south along the Irish Sea, past many beautiful sandy and pebbly beaches, secret coves and rockpools, over streams and along incredibly beautiful and breathtaking clifftops. We have many favourite beaches and places to paddle, play, fish and swim.

Cardigan Bay, and in particular our patch of Cardigan Bay, is home to the biggest pod of bottlenose dolphin in Europe, numbering over 300 animals. Spotting these dolphins can be a daily occurrence, although the lighter months, and especially the warmer summer months, are the best and most popular time to spot them. They grow to a length of about 4m (13ft), and in this area feed mostly on bass, mullet, salmon, sewin, garfish and mackerel. They are a most wonderful and magnificent thing to see.

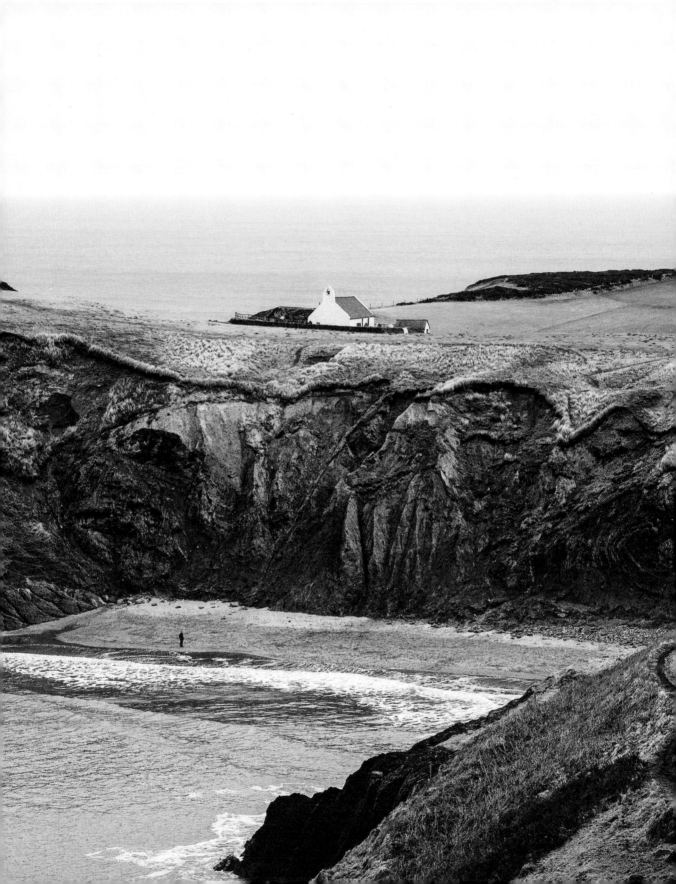

Beachcombing

Beachcombing involves searching the seashore for flotsam and jetsam, looking intently to see what interesting treasures the sea has washed ashore.

Walk slowly, walk mindfully. Take your time to contemplate all the little miracles of everything and enjoy your time exploring the beach. Hear the sea foam singing as the waves wash the tideline. Be soothed.

Whether sandy or rocky, every beach has its joys. Mostly I look for pretty little shells, smooth rounded sea glass, some textured driftwood and interesting pebbles — with holes through the middle (hag stones) or with stripes and crosses on the surface (often called wishing stones, you can skim or throw them back into the sea as you make a wish).

You may also find a gull's feather, or if you are lucky sharks' teeth, maybe some fossils, or a mermaid's purse (a brown leathery pouch with long curly tendrils that is a shark's or ray's egg case). Or maybe you will find a Victorian coin or some pieces of old pottery, a sea urchin skeleton, a dead starfish or little crab claws.

The more time you spend beachcombing, and the more things you look at, the more likely it is you will find what you're looking for.

The best time to go beachcombing is during the winter months or early in the morning when the beaches are empty. Go at a low or receding tide when there is more beach for you to savour and scour.

Right after a storm, when the rough seas have tussled the waters and shifted the sand and rocks around, is a very good time for beach bounty.

Of course, let us not forget that there is also, unfortunately, a great deal of rubbish washed up too. Sometimes interesting rubbish, fishermen's buoys and pots, for example, but mostly, just trash, plenty of plastic debris that we need to pick up and take away.

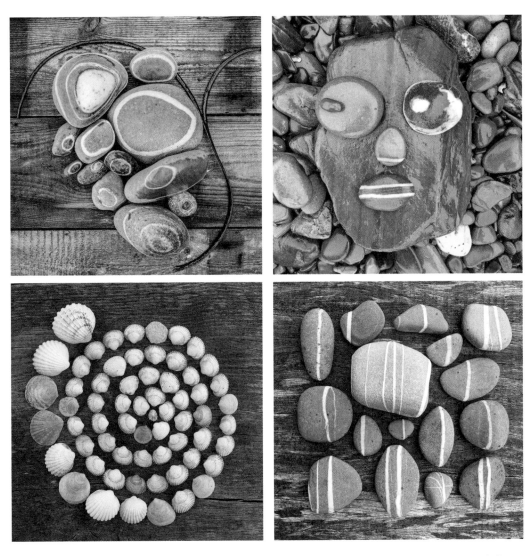

Stacking stones

Every little pebble in the stream
believes itself to be a precious stone.
Japanese proverb

Arranging pebbles or shells is meditative, totally absorbing, all-consuming and utterly calming. You become completely lost in concentration, absolutely and thoroughly busy. Walking the beach, eyes alert to find the right shape or colour, looking and seeing the different markings and patterns, wondering how a pebble got here, where it come from, about the passage of a pebble, thousands or even millions of years.

Many civilisations and cultures have placed spiritual symbols on rocks, considering them mystical silent beings. Holding a pebble in our hands connects us to an inclusive universe, to the continuous recycling, reshaping, making and reforming of the Earth's surface. A transient thing on a long journey, a pebble will have begun life as a much larger rock, millions of years previously, and will have been battered and washed before being found on the beach, at the bottom of the sea or at the river's edge.

I am not very good at balancing stones. I cannot create high towers or complicated structures, but that isn't really the point of this activity. It's the process itself that is so satisfying; it requires patience and focus to find the perfect balancing and resting points, to find harmony with the shapes and forms of your chosen stones. There is a deep stillness we get from just using the found and natural materials that surround us. It frees our minds of all other thoughts so that we feel grounded.

You will make your creations on a beach, on the edge of the ocean or by the running water of a stream or river surrounded by nature, and this is where you will leave them. They are temporary things and will return to their natural setting. Maybe in time, another person will come along and will hold these stones, look at them and build another tower. For me, this thought is both energising and comforting.

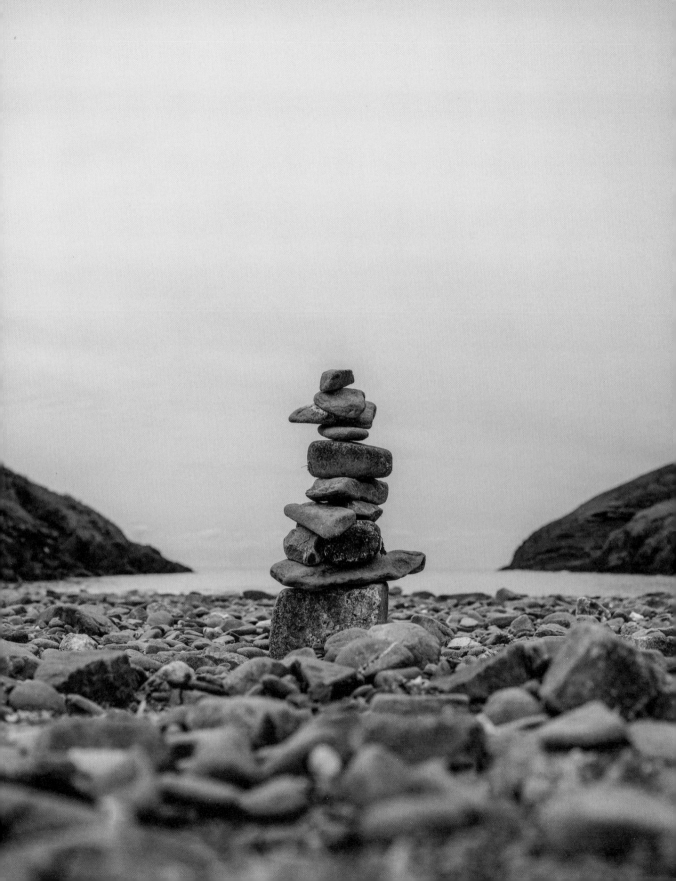

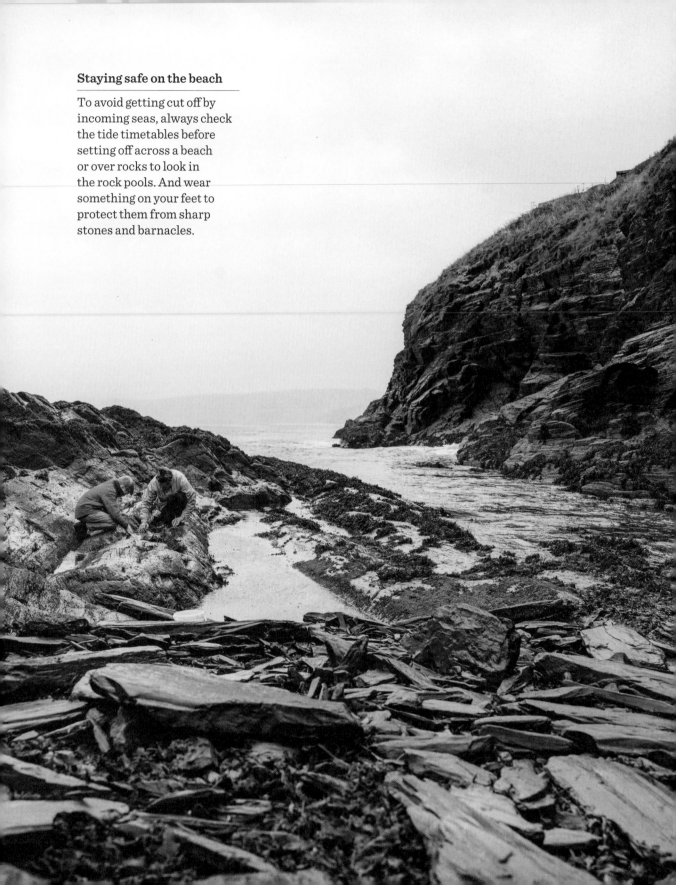

Staying safe on the beach

To avoid getting cut off by incoming seas, always check the tide timetables before setting off across a beach or over rocks to look in the rock pools. And wear something on your feet to protect them from sharp stones and barnacles.

Rock pooling

Rock pooling can lead to hours of absorbing discovery. When our four sons were younger much of our time by the seaside was spent looking into the rock pools: moving the seaweeds, peering into the crevasses, fascinated by the world of sea life and tiny creatures found living there.

How to rock pool

The lower the tide, the easier it is to find the more unusual creatures that lurk in the lowest part of the shore. Hiding beneath stones, around and between large boulders, stuck in tight crevasses, these creatures like to lie undisturbed where it is fairly shady, sheltered and safe.

It is best to pick up the creatures with your hands so as not to hurt them. Pick up crabs firmly but gently, placing a finger and thumb on the top and bottom of its body shell. Catch tiny shrimp and prawns in the cups of your hands, feel them flutter. Fast slippy and flippy fish are much harder to get.

Many sea creatures are well camouflaged and are very small. Lift the seaweed, look under rocks, be quiet, slow, careful and gentle. Look for crabs, mussels, shrimps, anemones, limpets, winkles, cockles, snails and starfish. Maybe you will find a mermaid's purse, the egg case of rays and sharks, which can vary in colour from a pale yellow, nut brown to black, with twirly tendrils on the end.

A clear bucket or container is always fun for a closer inspection, allowing you to observe the little creatures from all angles, moving, flitting, scuttling and swimming around. We usually put a bit of seaweed and a few pebbles in the bucket to make them feel a bit more at home.

Change the water regularly, though it is best to not keep them for long. Let them go where you found them.

Prawning and shrimping
Catch some eat some.

Most prawns caught in and around the UK are done so using lightweight plastic prawn pots. These are what Sean, the fisherman from our village, uses, mostly in the winter months, dropping them off into the sea from his small fishing boat. This style of fishing is very small scale, and pretty much all of his catch is exported live to Spain, where, like the spider crab, prawns are highly valued. Tragically, most of the prawns that we eat here in the UK are the larger farmed prawns from South east Asia. In this instance, though, bigger is not best. The prawns caught here are smallish, have rusty tiger streaks on their shells and taste so much sweeter and more delicious than farmed prawns.

When the time of the year and the tide is right, James often goes out across the beach with his net and walks into the shallows of the sea around the rocks to fish for prawns. There's no need for hooks, lines, tricky knots, bait, casting and reeling, you just need to push the net under the undercut nooks and crannies of the rocks and weeds to startle the prawns into jumping into your net. It sounds simple but, of course, like any fishing, it doesn't always come easy.

The best time to go prawning is when there is a calm sea at low tide, in fact, the lower the tide the better. As the tide goes out, prawns naturally come up towards the surface, making it easier to scoop them out of the water. Prawning is the perfect mixture of childhood fun, the joy of paddling and dipping a net into seawater mixed with the serious business of foraging for food for your table.

There is nothing better than taking prawns straight from the sea and throwing them into a pan of boiling water for a few minutes to cook. They need no accompaniment other than a nice glass of something chilled to wash them down.

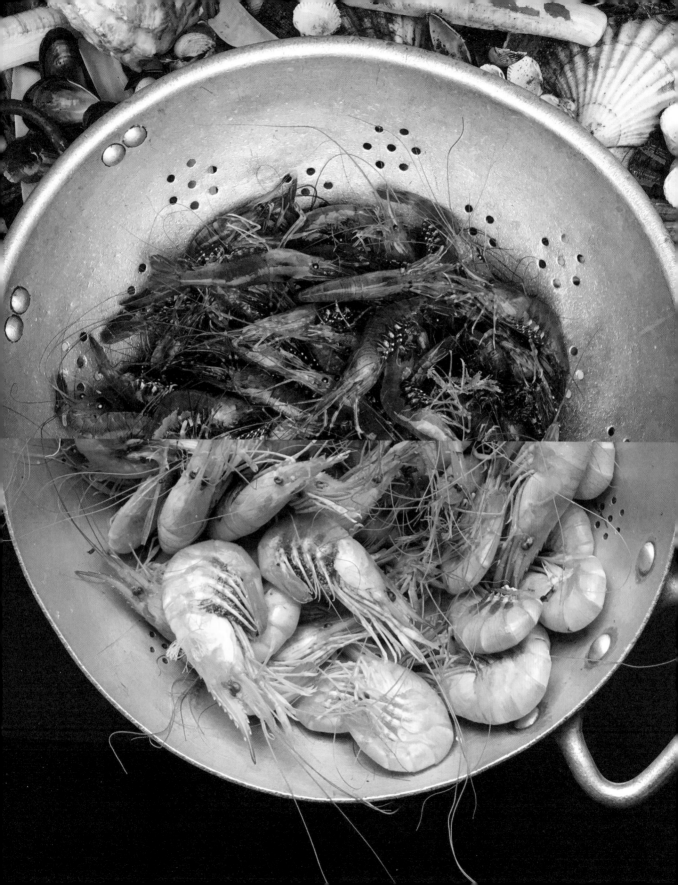

Catching razor clams

Razor clams are also known as razor shell, razorfish, the common razor or pod razor and, in Scotland, as spoots. In the US, there is a rounder Pacific version as well as the Atlantic one.

Common around the British coastline, and in Scandinavian waters and the Mediterranean, razor clams have a long rectangular shell, 10–20cm (4–8in) in length, that splits into two halves and resembles an old-fashioned cut-throat razor, hence their name. The shell is a sort of stripy light brown, grey to olive green, and it is quite brittle and fragile and it opens like a tall hinged door down the middle. The flesh of the razor clam inside is usually white to pale orange in colour.

Razor clams can be found in the low intertidal zone (seashore) of the sea. They rise out of their burrow to feed (when covered by the sea) by alternately expanding and elongating their 'foot'. To execute this trick, they need densely packed and firm silty sand that allows their foot to grip.

Although they need particular conditions, once established razor clams can be abundant. When the tide comes in and they are covered by seawater they feed by straining microscopic organic matter through their bodies. Then when the tide goes back out they dig down under the sand into their burrows to hide until the seawater comes back in again. They don't have eyes, instead they sense pressure changes and movements in the sand around them and, if threatened, can disappear in a matter of seconds. They grow in size during the summer, when it is warmer and there is a more plentiful supply of food. In winter they continue to feed but do not grow very much. On average, they increase in length by a few centimetres each year until they reach their maximum size of around 20cm (8in). They can live for up to 20 years.

Be patient and calm — for no one
can catch fish in anger.
Herbert Hoover

**Tips for catching
razor clams**

**Go down to the beach
on a very low cycle of a
spring tide** as that is when
the maximum amount of
the razor clam bed will
be uncovered. You must
walk slowly and carefully,
remembering the razor clams
will burrow down deep if
they feel threatened by the
change of pressure on the
sand. You need to look for a
little spout of water coming
out of the sand and a keyhole-
shaped hole.

**Have with you a container
of salt diluted with sea
water and a bucket.** When
you find a likely hole, pour
in a generous amount of the
salty solution, then wait a
few moments to see if the
clam comes to the surface.
The idea is that by squirting
the saltwater down the hole
will persuade the razor clam
to pop up, thinking it is high
tide and time to come out
and feed. When you do see
one pop out, gently but firmly
and very slowly pull it out of
the sand. Be very calm and
careful as grabbing it too
roughly will see it break up
and sink back into the hole.

**Cook them directly on the
barbecue.** When almost
ready the shell will pop open.
Carefully lift with tongs (or
oven gloves), as the shells
will be hot, and pour the
juice from each clam into a
saucepan in which you have
already melted butter and
sweated off crushed garlic.
Return each clam to the
barbecue, face down, for 10
seconds (a little charring
really brings out the flavour).
Add a big bunch of chopped
parsley to the sauce and very
quickly heat the mixture
through, though don't cook
the parsley. Put two or three
clams on each plate, pour the
sauce over and enjoy.

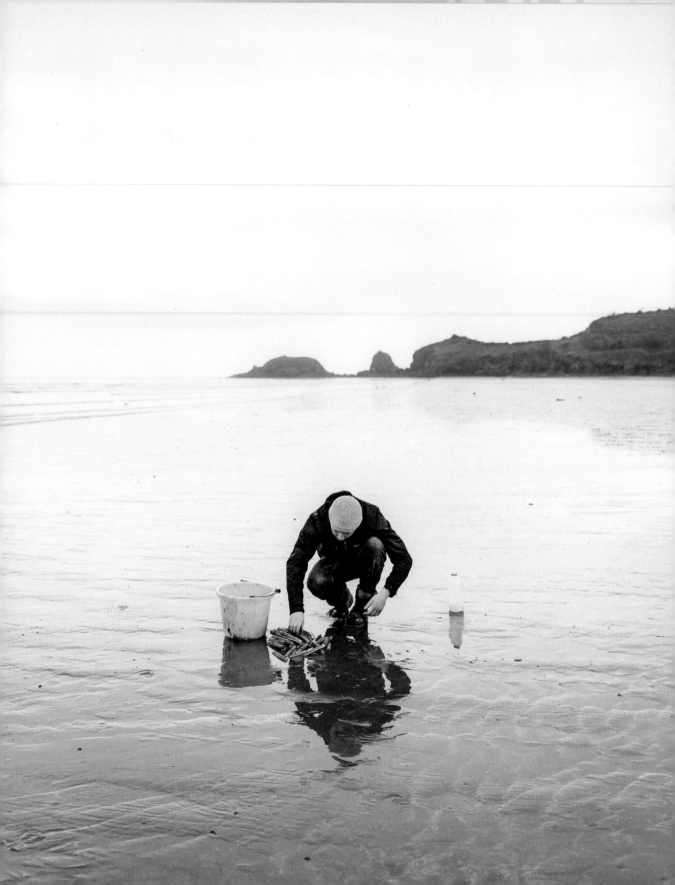

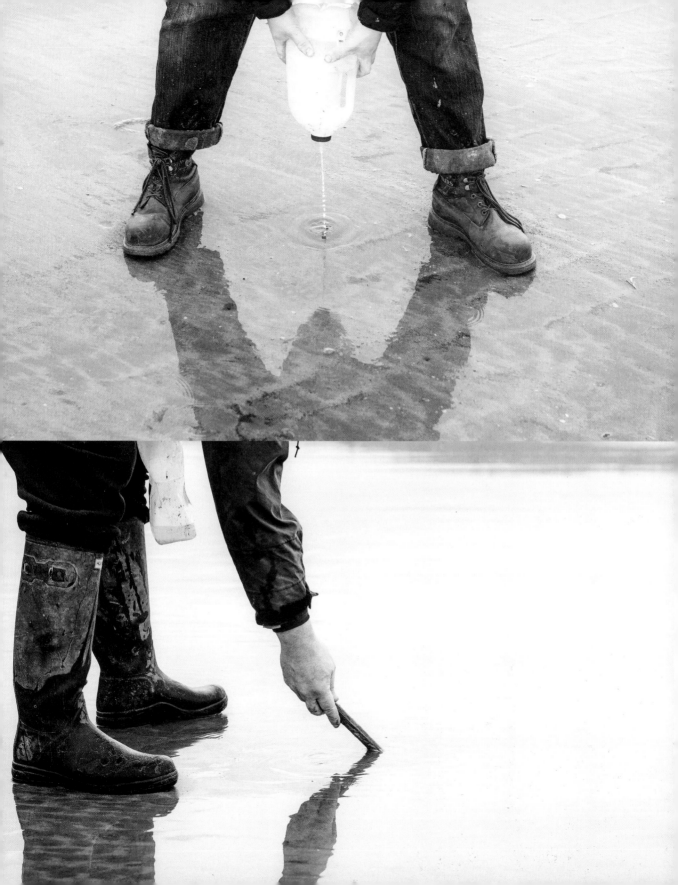

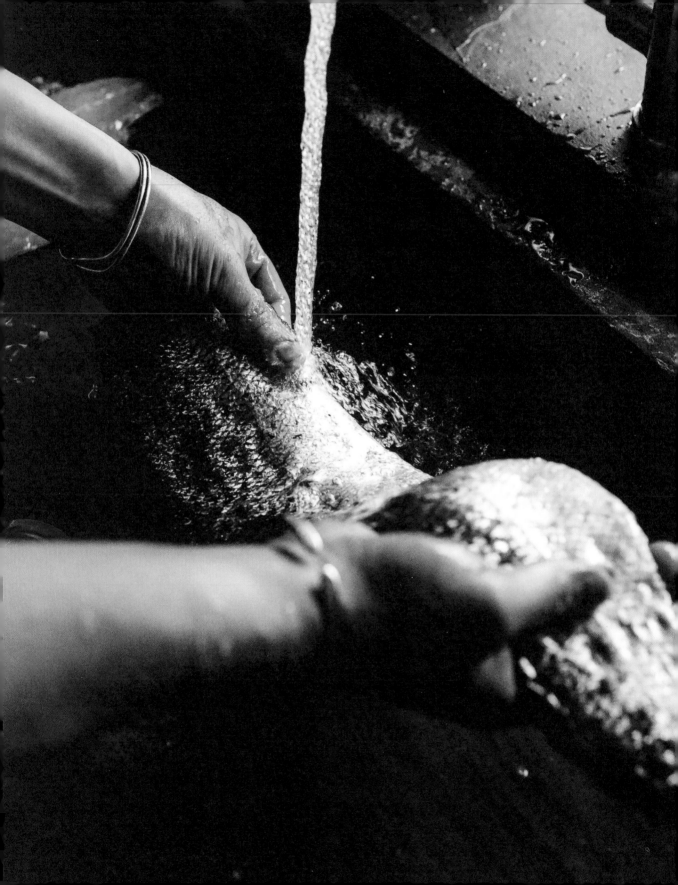

Salt-cured salmon
As told by James.

Curing fish with salt preserves it by reducing the amount of water in the flesh and so preventing harmful microorganisms from reproducing. This method of curing also firms up the flesh, giving it a better texture for presentation and slicing.

In the Nordic regions, where they have a fish-rich diet, they have sweet cures, saltier cures, aromatic cures, dry cures and wet cures, as well as many in-between ways of curing. My favourite, most tried-and-tested and preferred way of curing is as follows.

Ingredients

1 salmon fillet, skin on, cleaned and pin boned. For best results the fish has to be really, really fresh, the freshest you can get

approx. 400g salt. It is essential to use kosher salt or sea salt flakes. Don't bother using table salt as it will ruin the fish

approx. 200g soft brown sugar. Use two-thirds salt to one-third sugar. By adding sugar you will get a softer cure. For a firmer, denser fish cure use only salt

Method

Combine the salt and sugar in a bowl. Rub the mix all over the salmon. Place on a ceramic or stainless steel tray, cover with the remaining mixture, then clingfilm, and put in the refrigerator for 18 hours.

Scrape off all the salt mix then rinse the fish under running water, using a soft brush in the direction of the flesh to ensure everything is smoothed away. Pat dry with a clean tea towel, not kitchen paper as that will stick to the flesh. The fish can be served straight away, or wrapped in clingfilm and kept for a few days in the refrigerator.

To serve as sashimi, remove the skin (a skilled job but persevere) and then slice.

To cook, oil the skin well before placing skin-side down on a hot griddle, so it cooks slowly up through the skin. This way the skin will be crispy and the fish nice and moist when served.

Serve with boiled new potatoes, mixed while warm in a Scandi dressing made with the juice of half a lemon mixed with some crème fraîche, plenty of finely chopped fresh dill, a finely chopped small shallot and seasoned to taste with salt and pepper.

Catch a spider crab
As told by James.

Spider crabs are curious creatures. With their remarkably long legs, huge claws on the cock (male) crabs and prickled bright-red shells, their anatomy is as fascinating as their nature and habits.

In winter, they live in deep water, at depths of up to 120m (395ft), but in early summer, as water temperatures increase, they come closer inshore, to shed their shells and mate. Females can only mate in their soft-shelled state but once cocks are sexually mature they moult less often, maybe only every three or four years. Once a female has been fertilised she can remain stuck to the male for a week or two, I assume so the cock can protect them and his offspring while the female's shell hardens.

I avoid taking any female crabs, particularly when they're coupled, though it's not always obvious that this is the case. I have seen a nice big cock crab, dived down, grabbed it and started swimming back to the surface, only to find it's got a female underneath. Even when I let go, and the female drops out from the embrace mid-water, there is a sort of palpable desperation from the male to find the female and re-clasp itself. It seems to be more than instinct, it might even be love.

Plentiful and sustainable, up to 1,500 tons of spider crabs are landed around the British coastline each year, yet 95 per cent is whisked off to France and Spain, where they are valued as highly as lobster. Filter feeders and foragers rather than predators, spider crabs have white, sweet-tasting flesh.

Diving for spider crabs is always a fascinating adventure. There's a lot of pleasure in just the swimming. So much so that catching a crab seems like a bonus, even though it's actually the point. I do like the idea that you're foraging, that you're bringing something back for free, and that's a strong motivation. But it's the swimming in another world, a spellbinding, mysterious underwater world, that I find most rewarding.

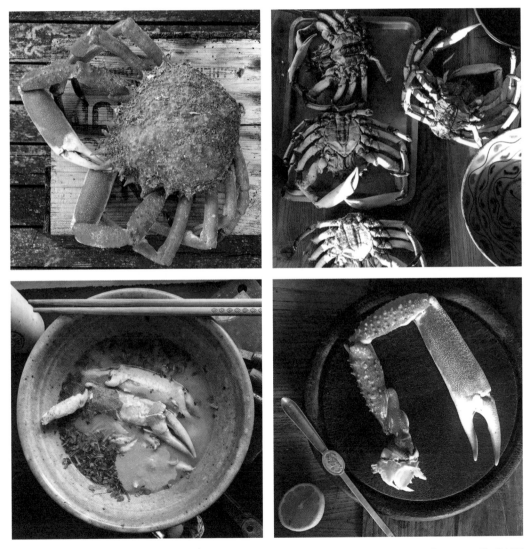

Seaweed

Seaweed is an ocean wonder, full of many minerals and nutrients.

About 70 per cent of the world's oxygen comes from seaweeds and microscopic algae. And seaweeds are amongst the fastest-growing organisms on the planet. They say that there are nine times more microscopic algae and seaweeds in the oceans than there are plants on land. Amazingly, seaweed absorbs minerals directly from the sea and is thought to be the single most nutritious food that you can eat.

Strictly speaking, seaweeds are not plants but algae, but, like all plants, they need sunlight for energy. The people of Japan and other Asian countries are famous for their love of seaweed, but across history many folk living near the sea have used and eaten seaweeds. The Vikings, Celts and Ancient Greeks all regularly ate edible seaweed for sustenance.

With intensive over-farming rapidly depleting our soil, we are beginning to look more and more to the sea as an especially abundant and rich source of healthy minerals to harvest. There are some brilliant small companies collecting seaweeds, so it is possible now to get hold of some fantastic dried seaweeds to eat.

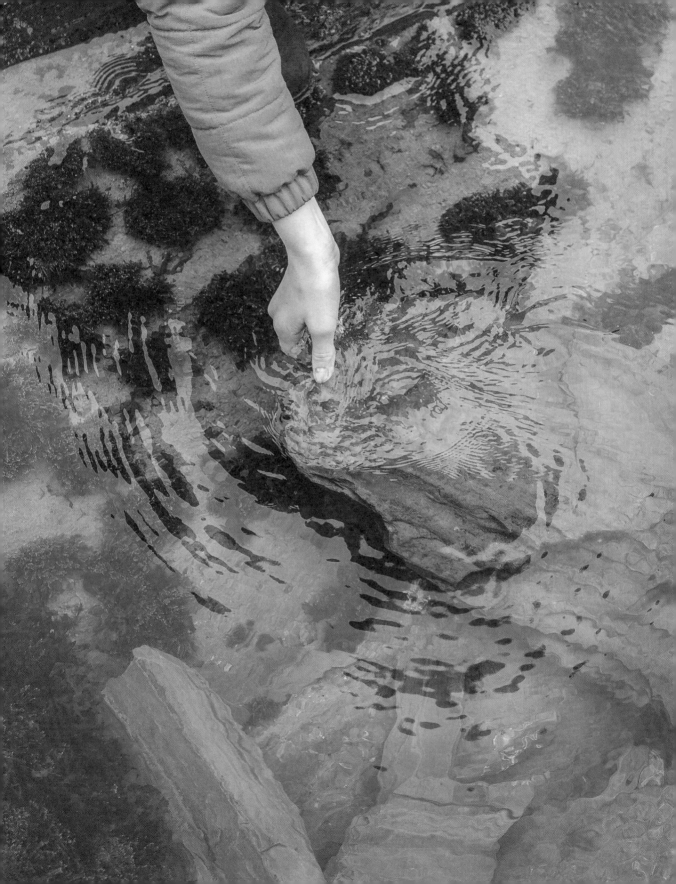

Types of seaweed

Bladderwrack is one of the best-known seaweeds. Its nutritional content varies seasonally; it is particularly high in vitamin A in the summer and in vitamin C in the autumn. Usually sold dried, it is found in traditional dishes in locations as far apart as Alaska and Japan. It tastes strongly of iodine, so is best used as seasoning in cooked dishes like stews or soups. Recognisable by its characteristic bladder-like air sacks on greeny-brown wavy fronds (which are a bit like bubble wrap and really fun to pop between your fingers), it's found all along our beaches in this part of West Wales.

Serrated wrack is the least edible of the brown seaweeds. Olive-brown in colour, it does not have air bladders, but flattened branching fronds with serrated edges. It has a very high iodine content, which gives a bitter taste, so it's not great to eat. If you put it in a hot bath, the high vitamin E content will cleanse and soften your skin beautifully. It also makes an excellent addition to your compost.

Gut weed is really bright green and grass like. It is found in rock pools and on the sand and mud on the shoreline. Tiny bubbles of air trapped inside its small tubes make it look a bit like intestines, hence its name. It is a good, easy seaweed to start off with, and it is pretty tasty too. After a thorough wash and dry, you can add some to an omelette or you can deep-fry for a couple of seconds to make it crispy, and season with equal amounts of salt and sugar.

Dulse is a dark browny-purple colour, thin and translucent like cellophane. Found growing off rocks in the cold waters of the northern hemisphere, it grows up to 30cm (1ft) long and can be harvested from late spring to autumn, though not, according to tradition, when there is an 'r' in the month. Iron-rich, it has a high mineral content (roughly ten times that of land vegetables). It also has a very high protein content and is low in fat. Loved by chefs, it has an umami richness that imparts a delicious savouriness to sauces, stews, rubs and marinades.

Carrageen is purple, with flat fronds up to 20cm (8in) long. Found easily on lower shore rocks, it is nutritionally rich in many vitamins and minerals. Widely found in Ireland, it was a source of trade for coastal communities there for centuries. In Irish folk medicine, it has been used to treat coughs, colds, sore throats and chest complaints, and it was also used as a home remedy for burns.

Sometimes called carrageen moss, it is widely used around the world, both fresh and hydrated, added to soups and stews as a vegetable. Its most common use, however, is as a gel that can be used to set or thicken liquids, often sweetened and flavoured to make jellies and desserts.

An exciting development in a medical research study showed the plant can slow down degenerative neurological diseases such as Parkinson's disease.

Laver is a fine, small, purple seaweed with broad, tough fronds. Found in the upper zone of rocky shores, it is one of the most commonly eaten seaweeds and is collected in Wales, Scotland and Ireland to make laverbread. Wales is famous for laverbread or *bara lawr*, which has nothing to do with bread so don't try looking for it in the bakery as my English friend did. After being boiled for 6 hours, laver turns it into something like a dark green purée, which is rolled with fine oatmeal into little cakes and fried into crisp patties. Enjoyed for a proper full Welsh breakfast with bacon, eggs, cockles and hot buttered toast, laverbread was said to improve the health of sick miners who suffered from gout.

Sea spaghetti is a long thin brown seaweed that not only looks like floating spaghetti but also can be cooked in the same way. We like to add it to any noodle dish, especially if we are eating fish. The tasty fronds make great broth as well. In France, Spain and Portugal sea spaghetti is commercially harvested and jarred in saltwater and lemon juice, then drained and used in salads and stir-fries. It is high in vitamin C and also phosphorus, which is thought to strengthen brain function.

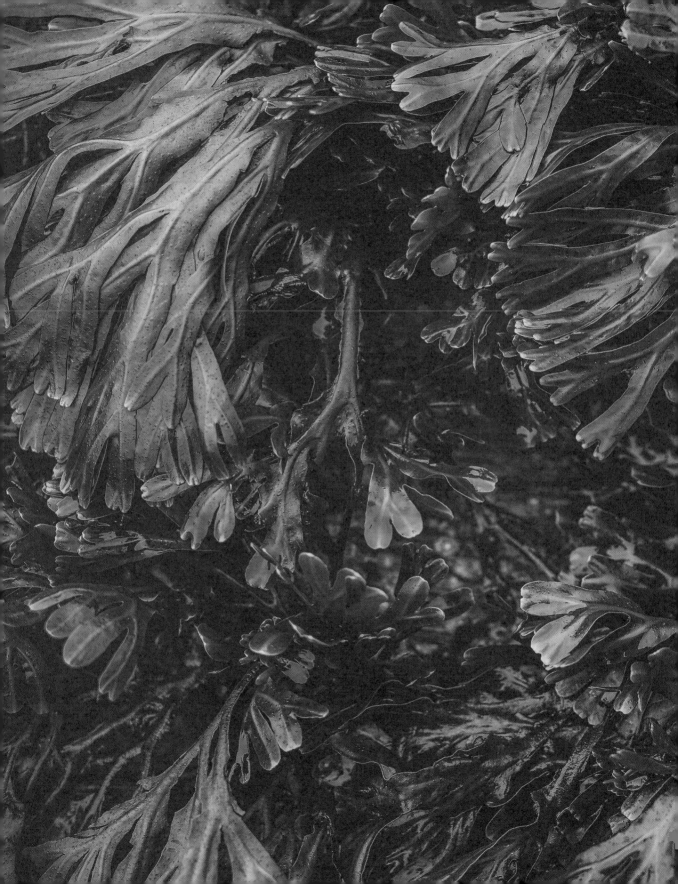

Seaweed butter

Seaweed and butter make for marine alchemy.

Our friend Max Jones, who is passionate both about all things dairy and fishing in the sea, comes to stay with us every now and then. He taught us how to make butter with the added bounty of the sea.

Use the freshest and best cream you can get, preferably organic cream straight out of a happy cow that has been milked to the sound of Bach playing in the dairy!

Ingredients

300ml (½ pint) double cream

collected and dried gut weed or 1 tablespoon store-bought dried mixed seaweed

good pinch of sea salt

Method

For fun, put the cream in a large glass jar with a lid and shake until it separates like Max would. You will know when it's ready as your arms will really ache, the cream will gradually become solid like butter and you will see buttermilk. Alternatively, you can whip it using a hand-held mixer and squeeze the rest of the batter out into a separate bowl.

When you think you have butter, transfer it to a sheet of greaseproof paper away from any heat. Mix the seaweed and salt into the butter until they are evenly distributed. Then pat your butter into shape. You can do this either by using greaseproof paper and your hands or wooden butter pats.

If you don't want the leftover buttermilk to go to waste, use it to make soda bread or scones.

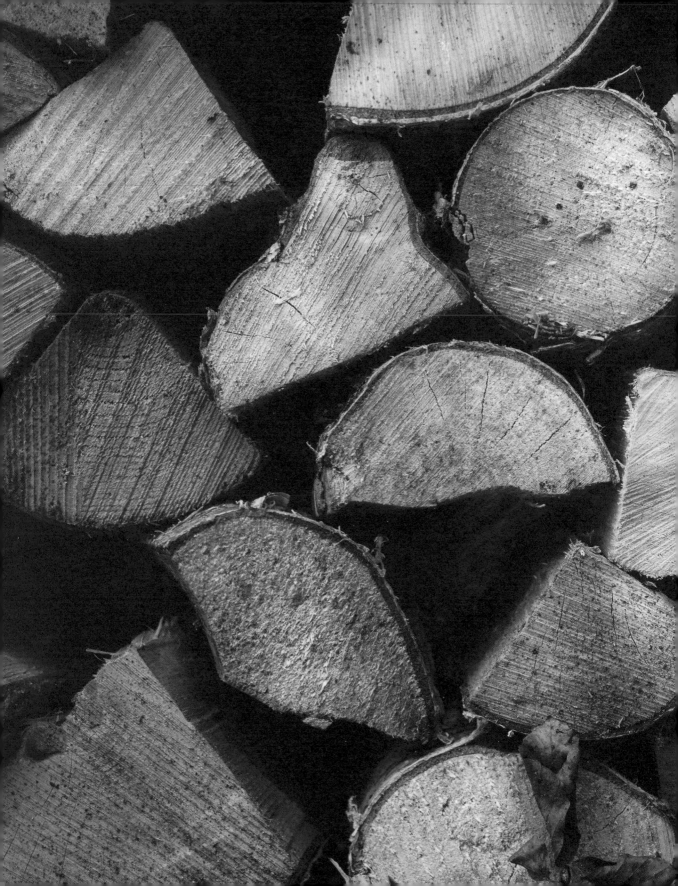

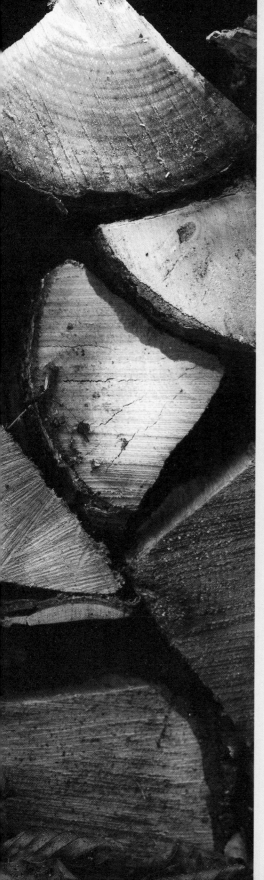

BY
THE
FIRE

The fire is the main comfort of the camp, whether in summer or winter, and is about as ample at one season as at another. It is as well for cheerfulness as for warmth and dryness.
Henry David Thoreau

Who isn't fascinated by fire? The flickering flames, the blaze of heat and the smouldering, smoking embers as it slowly dies.

When we first bought fforest farm we would frequently go there at the weekend and camp out with our boys, sometimes with friends. It was a time of figuring out exactly what we wanted to do. We would always start by building a fire, and the place that we always tended to build our campfire was where our big fire pit sits today. Since then, there has always been fire at fforest, from stoves for keeping the tents warm to smokers, barbeques and ovens for open-air cooking, as well as the big fire pit for talking and sharing stories, and a sing-song. Even our tiny stone pub isn't happy till the fire is roaring.

Fire is like the heart, it is a beautiful thing, bringing light with its sparkle and dancing flame. It draws us in around its warmth and glow, bringing community and conversation, calmly relaxing and uplifting our spirits, soothing our soul as we watch the fire crackling, flicking sparks of light that drift up into the night sky, reaching up to the moon and the stars above. The whiff of wood smoke wafting in the air heightens our senses, evoking primal memories and permeating into our clothes and hair.

Fire is a reward. Take pride and build it with care.

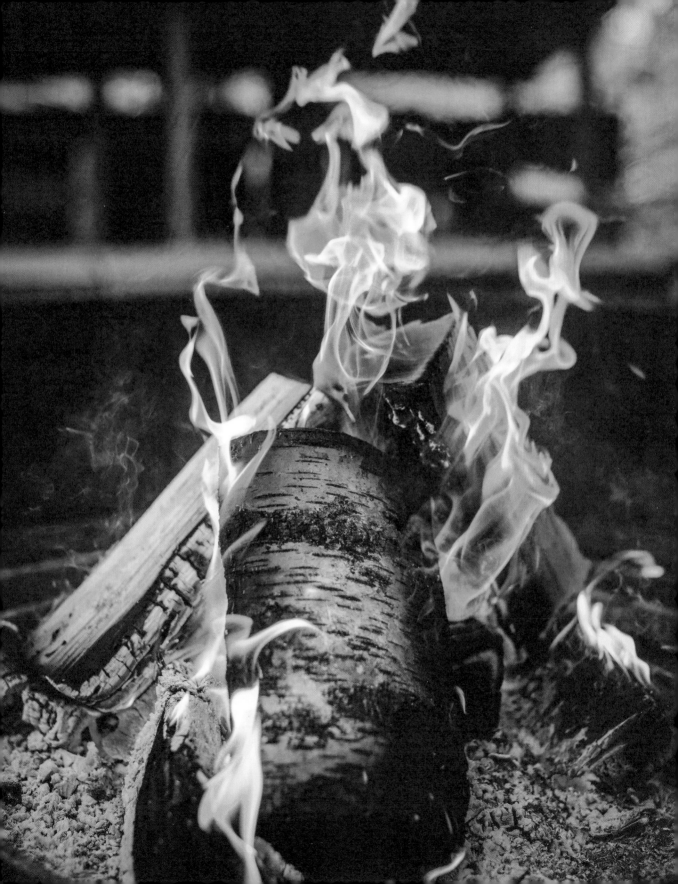

Chopping and stacking wood

The wood warmed me twice, once while I was splitting them, and again when they were on the fire, so that no fuel could give out more heat.
Henry David Thoreau

Being outside chopping, splitting and stacking wood for your fire is both immensely satisfying physically and mentally absorbing. There is the trance of concentration you can get into as you hold your axe high above your head to strike it down accurately onto the log, with just the right amount of force to split it.

Striking steady and with complete concentration, striking with rhythm. All this gives a huge sense of pleasure, watching the logs all pile up around you as you spilt and chop, followed by the repetitive action of stacking the logs neatly.

Tips for stacking wood

Take pride in your wood pile. Take pleasure in the sounds, the smell of fresh resin and sap, the tools, the stack.

Does your wood pile reflect your character? Are you an obsessive, measuring to make sure every log is cut to the same length? Are you a hoarder, storing wood in every nook and cranny of the garden? Are you an artist, creating a sculpture as you carefully consider where exactly each piece of wood will go? Or are you lazy, just tossing wood into the shed?

In northern countries and climates it used to be the case that having a good pile of wood stored up for the winter was a serious business — a matter of life and death, warmth or freezing, of having raw or cooked food. If people ran out of wood, they ran out of life. These days it is not such a matter of life and death to have a good wood pile but a huge amount of time and effort to this day is still put aside for the winter wood store.

Firewood must dry thoroughly before use. In the old days they wisely said that wood should be split before Easter so it can dry during spring and summer, ready for burning in the winter.

Bark, especially birch bark, slows the drying process, and split wood dries more easily than un-split wood. Dry wood does not go mouldy or rotten, and is much better for making a fire. If split wood is stacked bark-side up, the bark will act as a lid and slow down the drying process.

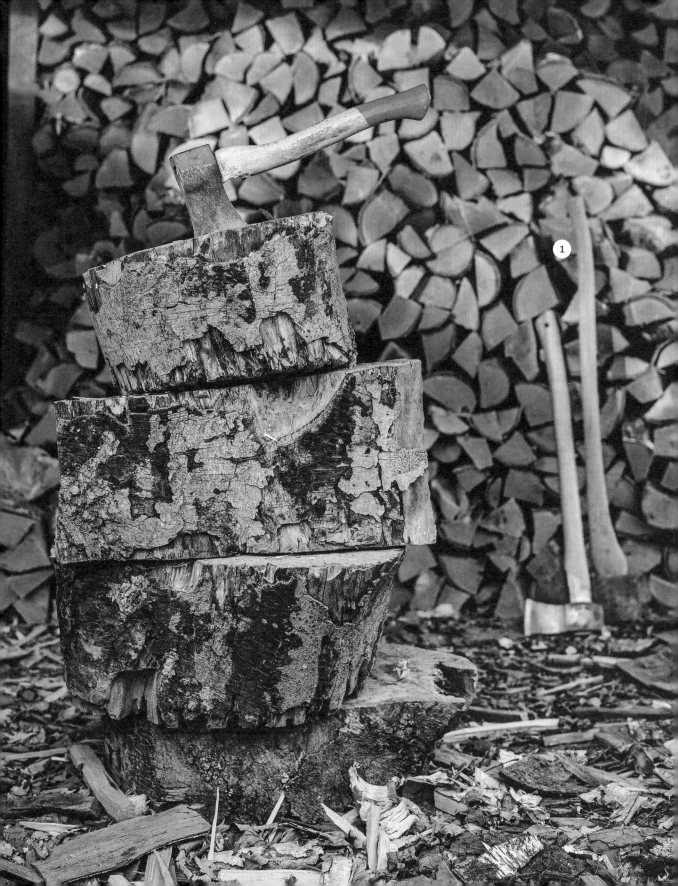

Types of axes

1

Felling axe (see page 167).
You don't often need one of these, these days, but for centuries it was the woodsman's most important tool as it is designed for chopping down trees. A felling axe is typically fairly light with a long handle, allowing the user to get good leverage and power into each swing. With the passing of time, this kind of axe, with its deep connection to forest life, has become obsolete.

2

Hatchet/carpenters axe.
These shorter-handled smaller axes are perfect for camping and small chopping jobs, like chopping kindling and wood for campfires.

3

Forest axe. This axe has a slim head and a slightly curved blade that allows you to cut across the fibres, cut across the grain of the wood. The head usually weighs about 1kg (2lb 4oz), and the handle is of medium length. (Just the one with the green string, see photo opposite). It is used for taking the limbs off branches and cutting small trees, not for wood splitting.

4

Splitting axe. As the name says, it is an axe for splitting wood.These axes have a large and heavy head that is wedge shaped, weighing from 1.3–1.6kg (3lb–3lb 6oz). It feels slightly front-heavy because it is balanced to cut directly downwards, quickly and easily splitting the wood along the grain. You are letting the sheer weight and momentum of the axe do the work, simply guiding the axe to where it needs to go.

5

Splitting maul. This is bigger, heavier and a more mighty tool than the splitting axe, although built in a similar way . Due to its size and weight, it is better for splitting bigger, thicker and knottier logs, which need a really hard knock to make them split.

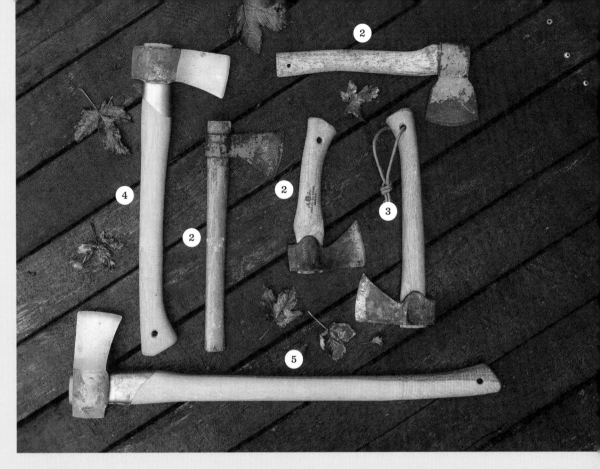

Axe safety

Make sure the head of your axe is secure, not at all wobbly, and the blade is always sharp.

Wear sturdy boots (no open toes!) and wear long trousers when you're chopping. These may not stop you from cutting yourself if your axe slips, but they can help reduce the seriousness of an injury.

A good chopping block is wide, heavy and flat at both ends. It should be completely solid and stable on the ground, not at all wobbly. A tree stump is ideal.

In the place you are working, create an 'axe area' where you're chopping, a safe zone of about 3m (10ft) around that people can't cross. And make sure you are not going to hit anything as you swing.

Stand square to your chopping block with your feet shoulder-width apart. Make sure neither of your legs is in front of the other, if you miss your target your front leg is the first place the axe will hit.

The safest way to pass an axe to someone else is to hold the handle near the end (called the knob) with the head down and pass it to them or lay it down so they can pick it up.

Always carry your axe with your hand under the head, with the sharp pointy bit turned away from your body.

Which wood burns best?
James gives advice on wood and charcoal.

What is the difference between hardwood and softwood? In general terms, hardwoods are any broad-leaved, deciduous trees, such as oak, beech and elm, while softwoods are conifers, including cedar and fir. Hardwoods are denser woods that burn hotter and longer than softwoods.

When it comes to burning wood in stoves, hardwood is better than softwood as it burns slower, but softer woods are easier to light and will produce heat faster. The density of softwood is around half that of hardwood, which results in it burning twice as fast — meaning you'll need twice as much!

Wood that hasn't been dried (seasoned) wastes much of the energy created while burning in removing water from the log and producing steam and corrosive tars that will clog and damage your flue. Fresh wood contains a high amount of water — between 65–90 per cent, depending on the species. It's best, therefore, if wood is seasoned for at least a year, preferably two, before burning. You can dry out your own wood in a wood store or, if you don't have the space, buy seasoned wood from a supplier. The best kiln-dried wood has a moisture content of less than 20 per cent.

For building a fire, use softwood kindling (such as birch-bark firelighters) for a fast flame to get the fire started, then add kiln-dried birch. Once the fire is burning hot you can add larger chunks of seasoned oak, which will reduce the airflow to the fire and produce a long and slow burn, which is ideal for keeping a stove going overnight.

Never ever burn scraps of construction timber in a stove or open fire. The preservative used in most construction timber (Tanalith) contains copper, chromium and arsenic. Similarly, board materials such as plywood and MDF are bonded with resins and formaldehyde. Burning such materials will release these elements into the air.

Woods for burning

Apple and cherry once seasoned well, are slow burning and wonderfully fragrant, so are great for cooking over.

Ash is a wonderful log for burning, lasting a long time and giving a steady fire and good heat, with virtually no smoke or spitting, even when burnt green (unseasoned), though it is always better to use seasoned wood

Beech burns similar to ash.

Birch is our preferred wood. The natural oils in the papery bark make it a natural firelighter that burns really hot. So always peel the thin top layer off to use for this purpose. Birch produces a strong heat but can burn quite quickly. It smells great too, but if cooking over it make sure all the bark is entirely burnt away as the deposits from the oils can taste bitter on the surface of any food cooked. Having said that, a little of the bark smoke can produce a spicy note in food, so experiment, but be warned that too much will ruin your dish.

Cedar is a light softwood with a wonderful smell that is popular for kindling as it has a high resin content. It lasts for some time and has a strong heat output, so take care not to overfill your stove. Cedar tends to crackle and spit a little. Its high resin content makes it very durable for its weight, which is why it is often used for external cladding and can be left untreated. We used it for cladding many of the buildings at fforest, and also, as it has antibacterial qualities, to line our showers and make our saunas.

Hawthorn/blackthorn is considered one of the best of the firewoods because it burns well with a steady flame and doesn't smoke much. It will burn slowly and hot for your wintery fires.

Horse chestnut produces a good flame and strong heat output but can spit, so is best kept for stoves.

Oak is the go-to wood for cooking with. The density of the wood produces a small flame, and when very well seasoned it burns slowly and steadily for a long time. Its embers also have a high heat and a long life. Sitting chunks of oak on the embers of charcoal and keeping it smouldering will produce smoke that will enhance the flavour of almost any food.

Pine is a softwood that burns well and smells festive. Try it for kindling or for outdoor fires.

Sycamore if seasoned well, will reward you with a good flame and moderate heat.

Pine-cone firelighters

The most common way to light a fire is to place scrunched-up balls of newspaper and torn-up egg boxes underneath your kindling, but at fforest we like, if possible, to use only natural tinder. Our preferred tinder is birch bark. It is an amazing fire starter, rich in resins, and peels off in a very satisfying way, like sheets of paper.

Another good tinder is cedar bark, which is extremely fibrous and resinous and can even be lit when damp. Pine needles, dried leaves and grasses, dead thistle heads, wood shavings, old man's beard and dried dock seedheads are all good options too, but they have to be really dry to work effectively.

Pine cones are very flammable and also make great firelighters. You can either collect them in the woods or buy them from garden shops or online.

Opposite is a way of making them even easier to light, which has the added benefit of using up the ends of your old candles too.

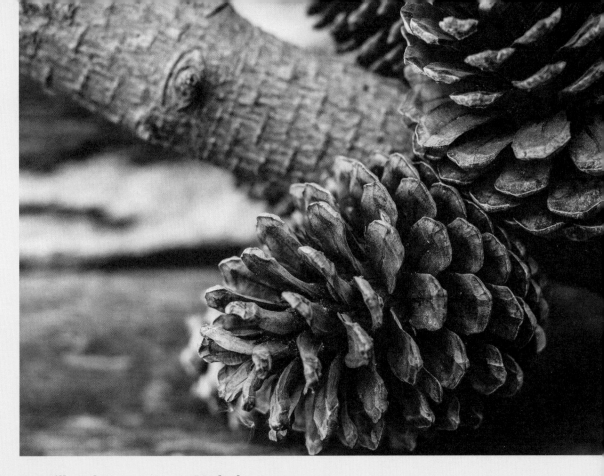

You will need

spoon

beeswax or soy wax from your old ends of candles, melted in an old clean saucepan over a gentle heat

some non-stick cupcake trays

candlewick or string to wrap around the base of your cones

pine cones

tongs for dipping the cones into the hot wax

sprigs of rosemary, lavender or pine needles (optional)

a few drops of wintery and spicy, essential oil, such as clove, mandarin or cinnamon

Method

Spoon the melted wax into the dips in the cupcake tray. Before placing each cone into the hot wax, wrap a length of candlewick or string around the base of each pine cone, leaving a little free to act as the wick. Using the tongs, carefully place each cone in a hole of the cupcake tray, making sure the loose piece of string is visible and ready for when you need to light it. At this point you could also add some sprigs of aromatic rosemary, lavender or pine needles if you like.

Leave to dry.

Once dry you can add a few drops of essential oil onto the pine cones.

Lift the pine cones out of the cupcake tin to store in a basket by the fire ready to use. Alternatively, package up for little gifts to give to friends.

Charcoal

The secret ingredient of the perfect barbecue is charcoal.

Charcoal is produced from burning or baking wood without oxygen in a form of kiln. All the moisture is driven out of the wood, together with other volatile components, leaving light carbonised wood or charcoal that, being free of water and tars, can burn at a much higher heat and also retain this heat for longer than wood. For this reason, charcoal is the traditional fuel of the blacksmith. Coke (baked coal) replaced charcoal in the commercial production of steel and iron during the Industrial Revolution. The best charcoal is made from seasoned hardwoods. At fforest, we have two or three sources of charcoal. Two are local and traditional, the other is commercially produced. It's a good product, but we tend to use this only when our local supplies are exhausted.

People have been making charcoal for thousands of years, since about 4000 BC. Charcoal was used primarily for fires, particularly in medieval times, because it burns hotter and cleaner than wood, and is less smoky. It also burns more slowly, making it especially good for melting metals such as copper, tin ore and bronze.

Most folk now commonly use charcoal for cooking outdoors, as we do here at fforest. We are very lucky that our neighbours who run a coppice wood also make charcoal, and it is from them that we obtain our charcoal. Hardwoods such as oak and beech are the best to use as they have a very slow burn.

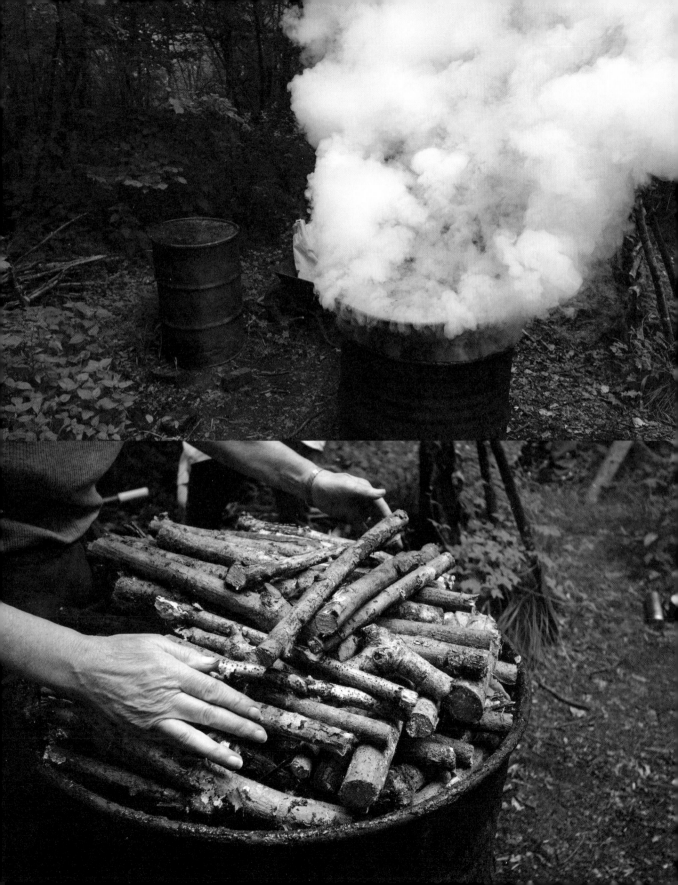

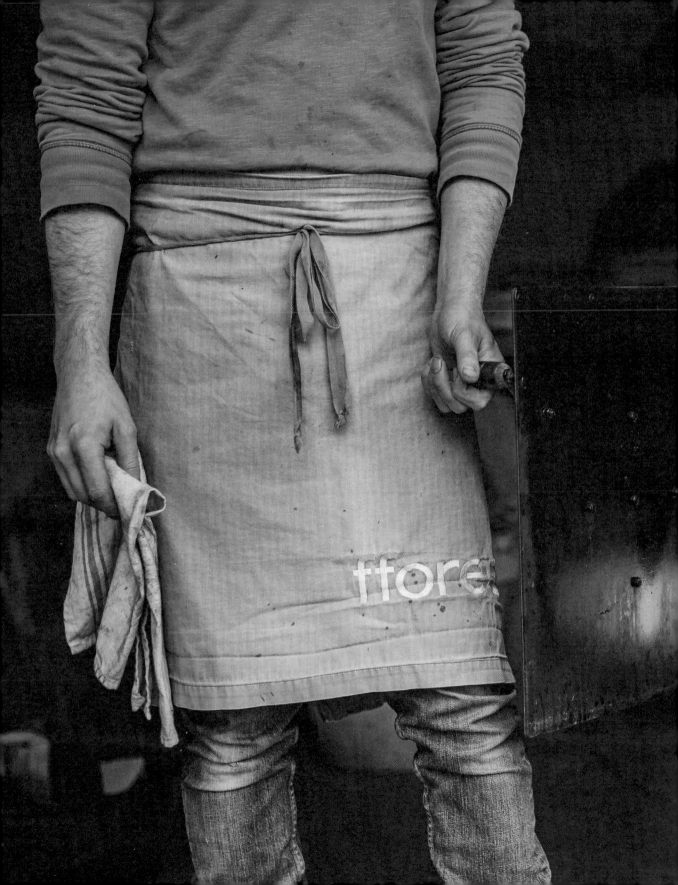

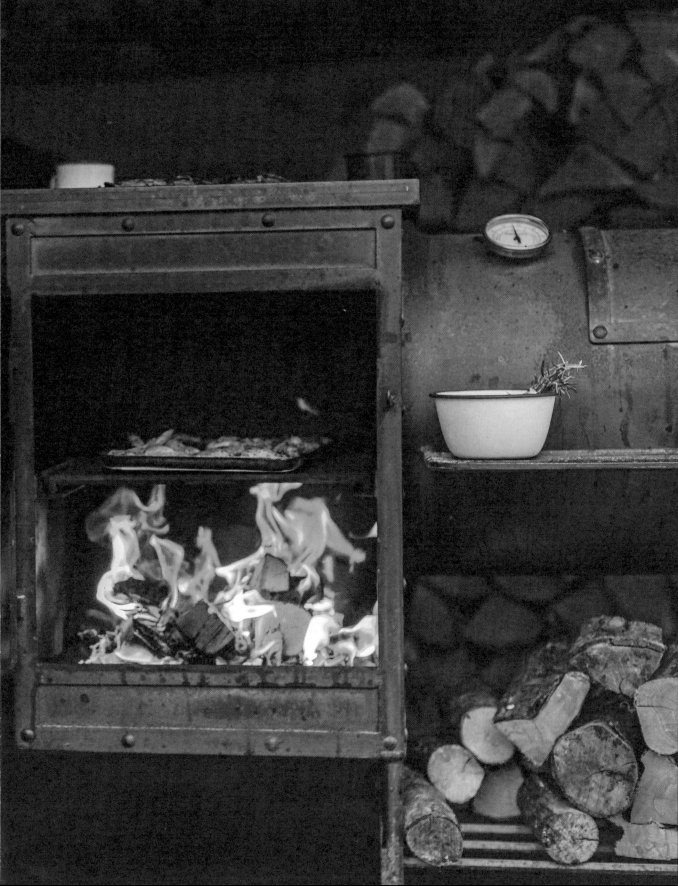

Barbecuing

Gathering around food, community, sharing and talking are all very important to us, and cooking and eating in the great outdoors offers great rewards.

The elemental nature of cooking over fire is always a pleasure. Cooking over charcoal is easier than cooking over wood but the higher temperature has to be understood and managed.

The barbecue

Don't be afraid to improvise. Dustbin lids, shopping baskets and steel buckets can all be pressed into service. My home barbecue is a cast-iron sheep trough (great for holding heat) — it is the one I most often use at fforest and it is more than 20 years old. I had it made for a big barbecue at the kids' school. It is stainless steel, weighs too much, has become contorted with the heat over the years, but we are old buddies. It doesn't let me down.

The implements

welding gauntlets

2 broad, long-bladed stainless steel burger flippers

2 pairs of stainless steel tongs

Welding gauntlets are essential, cheap and make sure you don't burn yourself. The flippers are for the lifting and turning. If you're cooking large pieces of meat, pairs of these flippers and tongs help a lot.

When turning large pieces, always take the griddle off the barbecue and put it on a flat baking tray. You can then take it easy without the heat and get to all sides.

Lighting the barbecue

Make a pyramid of kindling against the back of your barbecue. Once the little fire is burning well, put your charcoal in, heaped around and against the sides of the fire, but don't cover it or you will put it out. Ensure all your bits of charcoal are huddled together, without stragglers. Leave for 30–40 minutes, without prodding or spreading until the charcoal is bright red and very hot. At this point you can spread the charcoal into an even layer and put your grills on. In around 15 minutes or so the charcoal will have turned white on top with the body still glowing beneath. That's when it's ready to cook.

fforest barbecued whole boned chicken

If you have ever been to fforest, chances are you will have eaten this at least once during your stay. For some people it's the only reason they come.

Ingredients

1x 2.2kg (5lb) free-range chicken. Get your butcher to bone it out, but keep the chicken whole, effectively like a butterfly. Retain the bones and use to make a chicken stock for another day.

For the marinade

1 large juicy lemon, juice and zest

1 large garlic clove, crushed

plenty of fresh garden herbs, such as rosemary, thyme, parsley, tarragon, finely chopped

sea salt

freshly ground pepper

a good few glugs of olive oil

Method

Mix together the marinade ingredients and rub into and all over the chicken. Leave in the refrigerator for a good few hours, ideally overnight.

Light the barbecue 45 minutes–1 hour before you intend to cook on it and preheat your oven to 140°C (275°F), Gas Mark 1.

Place the chicken in an oven proof dish and place in the oven for 45 minutes — you're looking to get the internal temperature up, not to cook the chicken — then remove from the oven and finish on the barbecue.

Check the heat by holding your palm flat out a couple of centimetres above the grill. If you can hold it there for 5 seconds you are ready to cook. Any less, wait.

Before you start cooking, put on your welding gauntlets, take off the grills and oil them to prevent the chicken from sticking to the grill.

Open up the chicken and place flat, skin-side up, on the grill and cook for about 25 minutes, until a good colour but not to burnt. When you are happy with the colour, flip to cook the other side.

Trust your judgement and refrain from moving the chicken too much as this can cause you to cut the skin. The best tool for moving the chicken is a long fish slice, which is great for getting underneath the whole chicken so you can move it around all in one piece.

To check your chicken is cooked, cut into the largest area of breast to see if the juices are running clear. If done, remove from the grill and leave to rest for a few minutes.

Slice the chicken, ready to serve, and put it back into any cooked tasty marinade juices.

Campfires

Who has smelled the woodsmoke at twilight, who has seen the campfire burning, who is quick to read the noises of the night?
Rudyard Kipling

There is a ritual to building a fire. There is a way of doing it that is about keeping a connection with the place, but we only have one rule: no firelighters. At least, nothing we can't scavenge from the fields and woods.

How to build a fire

Begin by gathering the tinder, not paper if you can avoid it. The satisfaction lies in building something entirely natural within its surroundings. Our preference is for what we call 'the magic stuff'—dried seedheads or stems, and what we had plenty of when first at fforest: dock stems. We would also collect more than we needed and store them.

Then the twigs: look up into the trees and you will see branches still attached, but dead and dried out, some quite fine, some quite big. The larger ones will be easy to snap off, but take care not to damage the live part of the tree or bush. Don't be tempted by branches on the ground.

Even in a dry summer, these will have absorbed moisture from the ground and will be impossible to light until the fire is established. You will need twigs of matchstick thickness, pencil thickness, and finger thickness.

To start your fire, create a dry base make a 'raft' of the finger-thick twigs laid side by side, about 15–20cm (6–8in) square. Then lay a mat of your tinder, and on top of this layer, your matchstick twigs, crossed over 'jenga style', working from the outside in and leaving a 5cm (2in) open funnel in the middle. Take your pencil sticks and build a tipi shape over the jenga stack, with the feet touching the mat below. Leave a door

into the tipi, facing the wind, then repeat the tipi structure with some more of the finger-thick twigs.

Take a small ball of tinder, light carefully, sheltered from any wind. Once the flame has taken, gently push it through the door of the tipi to the centre of the fire. You can assist the flame by gently blowing or use an elder fire stick to direct oxygen to the heart of the fire.

Once the flame is established, build up the tipi shape by adding larger and larger pieces. When there is sufficient heat, green or damper wood can be added, although this will always make your fire smoke more.

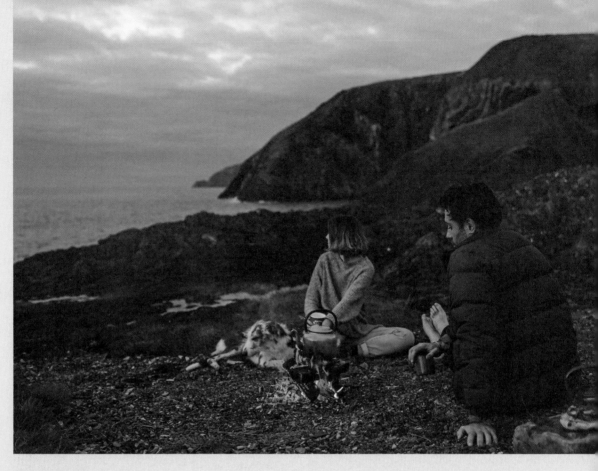

Keeping safe

An open campfire provides essential light, wonderful warmth and a place to cook. However, if not treated with care, fires can quickly become dangerous and pose a risk to both people and the environment. Always treat a fire with respect and obey the following rules:

Never burn anything other than wood on the fire.

Store extra wood away from the fire.

Indoors or out — never leave your fire unattended.

Keep fires small, they are better for cooking and use less fuel.

If you are having a fire outside, always check you are allowed to have a fire.

Choose a clear area, away from trees and bushes, and from overhanging branches.

Make a circle of stones around it.

Keep a bucket of water or sand to hand in case the fire gets out of control.

Always put your fire out before you leave and, if you have a fire in the wild, ensure you leave no trace of having been there.

Campfire bread

This comes from the pizza dough recipe used at our pizza restaurant, Pizzatipi, in Cardigan. The recipe has been tweaked over and over by our sons. It can be rolled out or flattened by hand. It makes 6 flatbreads.

Ingredients

220ml (8fl oz) lukewarm water

2g (0.07oz) dry yeast

367g (12½oz) flour (00 flour is best but you can use half strong and half plain), plus extra for dusting

13g (½oz) fine salt

Method

Mix the water and yeast together in a large bowl until the yeast has fully dissolved.

Add the flour and mix until partially bound (torn up and messy).

Add the salt (salt kills yeast, so we want the water and yeast to come into contact with the flour first). Mix until it starts to become smooth, waiting until it looks right.

Turn out onto a table and knead until the dough is silky smooth.

Chop into 6 pieces (about 100g each (3½oz). Turn into tight but smooth balls by folding the outside into the middle.

Leave on a tray for 6 hours to rise or in the refrigerator for up to 48 hours for maximum flavour.

When ready to cook, flour your hands and tease the dough balls from the tray (it is best to use a dough scraper to scoop them out and to keep the shape, but clean bank cards help do a good job). Using lots of flour, either roll out or flatten the dough using your fingers/hands/elbows.

Shake off any excess flour and pop on glowing coals or, even better, a griddle pan over coals, and cook until almost charred on each side.

Campfire popcorn

Everyone loves popcorn, especially kids, and making it over a fire is both fun and easy to do.

Method

Take two matching metal bowl sieves, making sure they both have a loop of metal at the top end to be able to hinge the two sieves securely together. Join the sieves together with a piece of wire, making sure that you leave enough flexibility to open and close them.

Then use more wire to lash one of the handles to a longer stick or pole so you can put it over the fire without burning your hands.

When you are ready to go, add a handful of corn kernels into the bottom of the sieve basket, close the top down and secure closed. Hold the basket over your fire and let the popping begin. It all happens very quickly and is really a fun thing to see. When the corn has all popped, wait a few moments for the metal to cool down before carefully opening the sieves.

You can add either a little sprinkle of salt or sugar as you prefer, before doing it all over again.

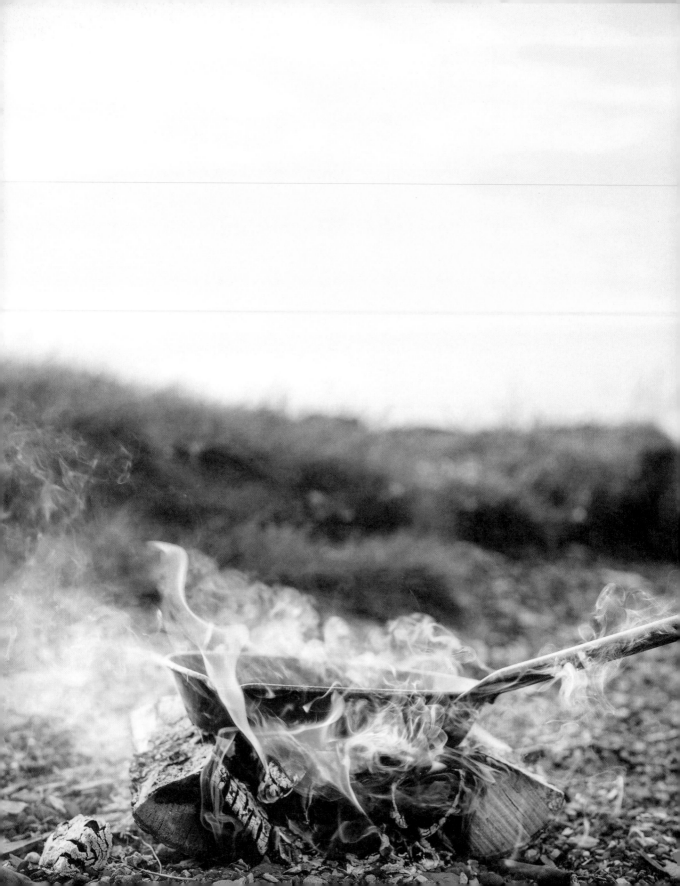

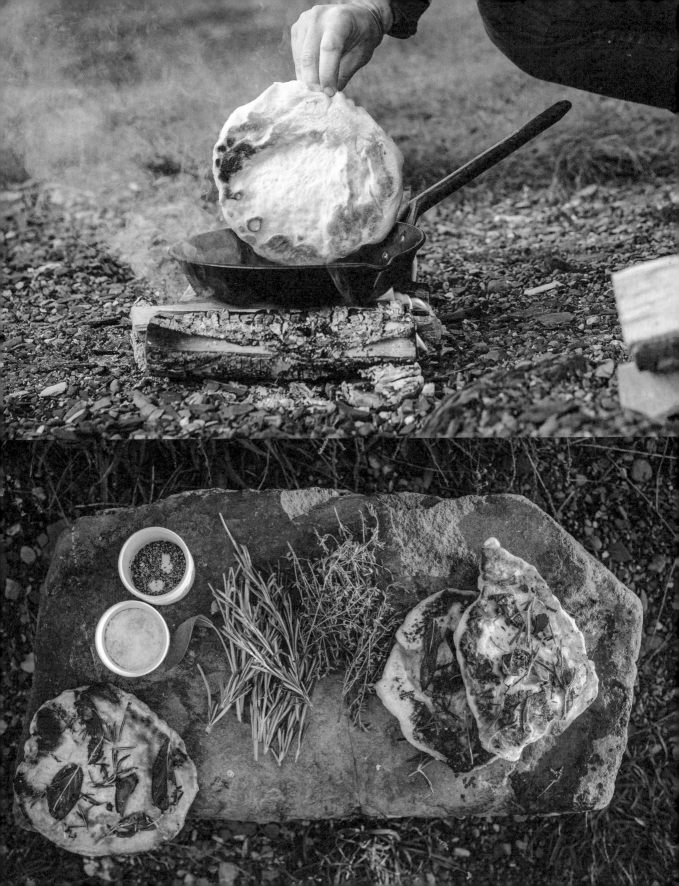

Fireside games, warmth and talking
Life is more fun if you play games.
Roald Dahl

Fire is a reward. It draws you in, offering light, warmth, community and conversation. Watching the flames dance and flicker, soaking up the heat and the smell of the woodsmoke encourages us to share stories, talk and exercise our lungs with laughter, to be warmed by the company of friends, maybe sing some songs or play some games.

Campfire yells, chants and cheers are a way to let off steam, to get moving, shaking and singing. Who doesn't love a sing along, and how good it makes us feel? Singing is so uplifting, it's something we should make more time for. It brings fun to the day, makes us happy, makes us laugh and completely improves our mood.

Anytime, of course, is good for playing games, a rainy day inside, or a sunny day outside. Here are some of our favourites:

Campfire games

nature treasure hunt

arm-wrestling

dictionary game

consequences

throw the smile

forehead detective

charades

truth or dare

Nos da — as we say in Wales — or good night. And sleep well, with sweet and happy dreams.

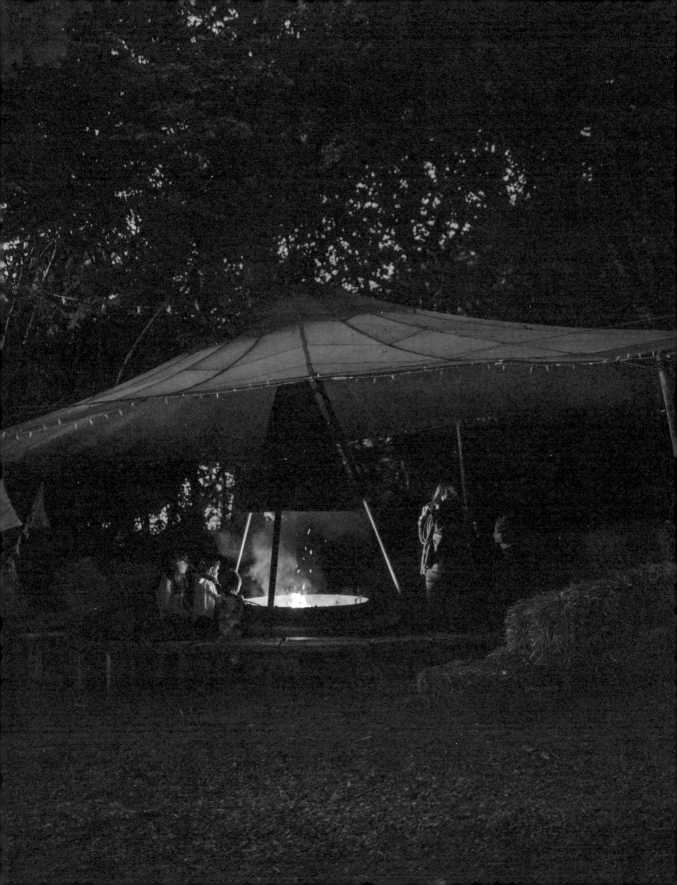

Index

Acknowledgements

Thank you Judith Hannam for your patience, calm and gentle nudging from start to finish. Thank you to Isabel and all at Kyle Books for believing in this book and making it happen.

Very special thanks to Nick and Harriet Hand at The Department of Small Works for your wonderful friendship, laughter, help, guidance, design and incredible attention to all the little details, I really could not have done this book without you.

Huge thanks to Finn Beales who took all the beautiful photos in this book and who was so calm, a total dream to work with. And thank you Clare, Harlan and Seren for making it so much fun.

Thank you to Nick Hand for taking the photos for the endpapers, also thank you Nick and Ellen at The Letterpress Collective in Bristol, for creating and printing the woodblock type for the cover and the chapter headings, they are a perfect addition.

Thank you to Richard, Sarah and Eli King, Leah and Jim Parkyn, Caryl and Phil, Gordon and Belinda Stovin, Beccy and Jon, Holly Bath, Max Jones, Reidin Beattie, Kate Dunwell, Jac and Fliss, Rowan, Tamsin, Brook, Heather, Ali clifford, Lillie O'Brien, Anja, The Herberts, Dia Crabs, Lizzie Everard, Judith Rees, Tess, Rae and Emily for all your help, advise, kindness and encouragement through out.

A heartfelt thank you to everyone who works at fforest and who has worked at fforest, you have kept our dream gleaming and strong with your tireless efforts and warm smiles every day.

Very special thanks and hugs to Amanda who holds us all together and Bronwen for all the tiny, little details.

Enormous gratitude to everyone who has been to stay at fforest over all the years.

We have met so many wonderful people who have become such good friends and have become part of the fforest community. You continue to inspire and energise us and all bring such pleasure, warmth and contribution. Very big thanks to everyone who has shared so much with us at Gather, Glow, feast and all the other events. There are too many to mention individually, a massive thanks to you all.

Warm thanks to all the wonderful instagram connections I have made on @coldatnight and @fforest I really relish these daily interactions and love when we meet for real.

Last but not least the biggest love to my incredible family and partners on this journey, James, Jackson, Robbie, Calder and Teifi, you are my world and inspiration. Huge love to my parents, Jann and Tony also to my dearest sister Amanda.

Hugs to all our fforest dogs Bru and Arrow, Shrimp and Mossy x

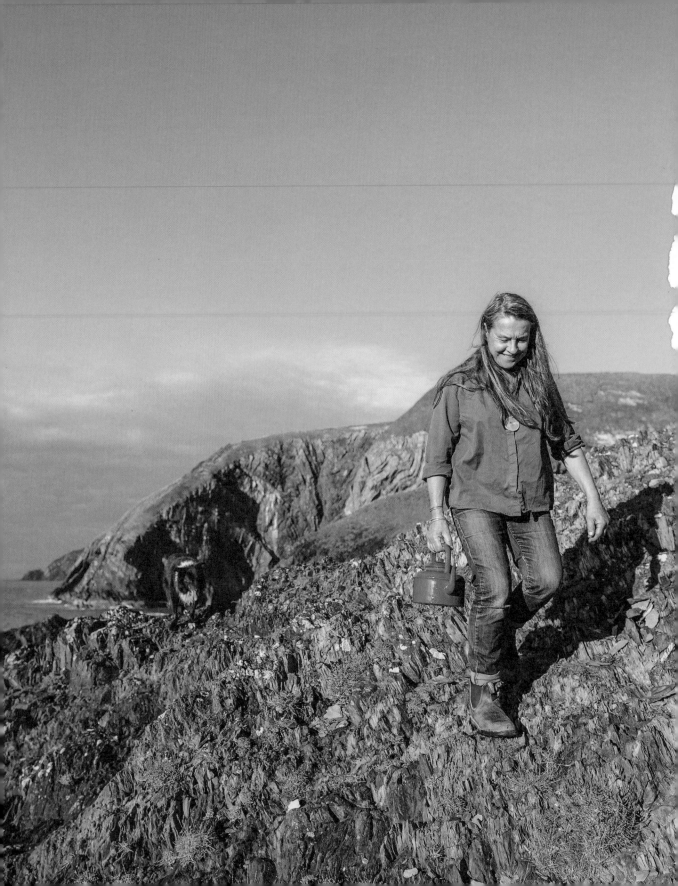

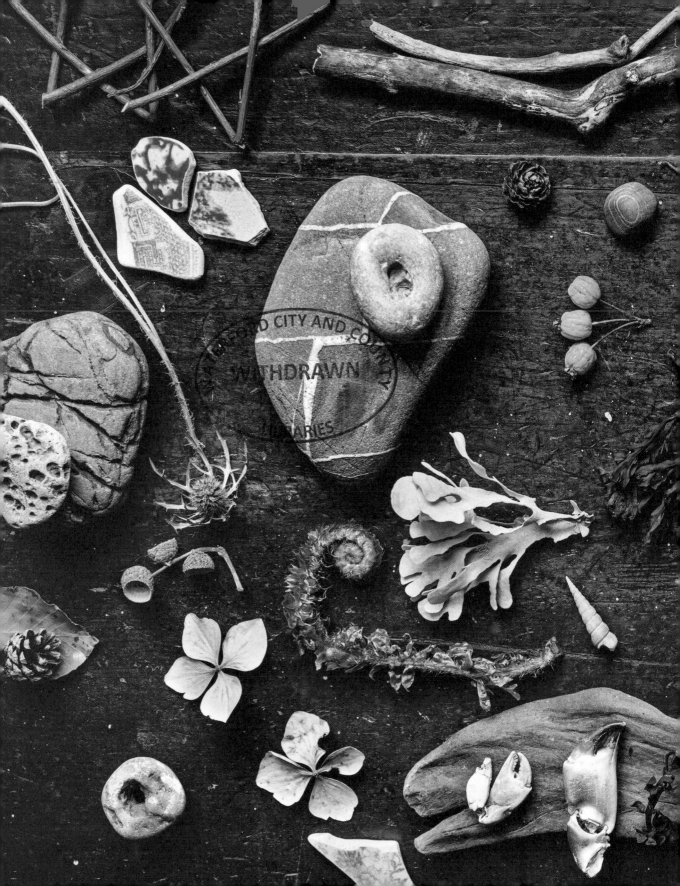